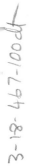

THE PHYSICIAN
AND COST CONTROL

The Physician and Cost Control

RA410.53
P47

Edited by

Edward J. Carels
Comprehensive Care Corporation

Duncan Neuhauser
School of Medicine
Case Western Reserve University

William B. Stason
Harvard School of Public Health

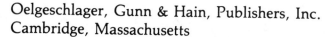 Oelgeschlager, Gunn & Hain, Publishers, Inc.
Cambridge, Massachusetts

International Standard Book Number: 0-89946-005-4

Library of Congress Catalog Card Number: 79-21736

Printed in the United States of America

Library of Congress Cataloging in Publication Data
Main entry under title:

The Physician and cost control.

Based on a conference sponsored by Harvard School of Public Health, Center for the Analysis of Health Practices, and others, held Dec. 9-10, 1978.
Includes index.
1. Medical care—United States—Cost control—Congresses. 2. Physicians—United States—Congresses. 3. Medicine—Practice—United States—Congresses. 4. Medicine, Clinical—Decision making—Congresses.. I. Carels, Edward J. II. Neuhauser, Duncan. III. Stason, William B. IV. Harvard University. Center for the Analysis of Health Practices.
RA410.53.P47   658.1'514   79-21736
ISBN 0-89946-005-4

Contents

List of Figures

List of Tables

Foreword:
Remarks at the Conference on
the Physician and Cost Control

Our presence here this morning is symptomatic of a national pre-occupation—obsession almost—with health, health care, and the costs of buying the latter in pursuit of the former. It is true that some authoritative figures are indifferent to a health budget upward of $160 billion per year and rising rapidly. For them, the size of the health care establishment and its capacity to employ workers of all levels of skill makes it a model public work. Most of us feel, with Emerson, however, that events are in the saddle and ride mankind, that the system is out of control, and that we stand to lose much that is good in other spheres of public life, areas in which public investment is jeopardized by our appetite for health-related resources. Hence this conference on cost control.

Although there are surely large-scale forces influencing the economic behavior of the health industry, it is almost unique among organized activities of its size in the dispersion of the authority to make decisions about the use of resources. Those decision makers are, of course, physicians. And so it is that the organizers of this conference have elected to focus the proceedings on our behavior as practitioners and to ask whether, and perhaps how, our decisions about the allocation of resources might continue to serve the perceived needs of patients as well as serve better the perceived social needs to contain costs.

It is unfortunate that cost control in the medical sector is not a policy issue in the sense that it provokes widespread discussion of lofty goals, and the rhetoric and emotional commitment of the Crusades. Most of us grew up professionally during an area in which it was much easier, and more fun, to simply bring in more money by the front door than to try to stop it from going out the back. But even if cost containment is not truly a policy issue, some resolution of the problem seems to be a necessary preliminary that must be gotten out of the way before other issues can be realistically discussed.

Practical, local approaches to cost control are the products we hope this conference will achieve. Success will result from, not only your efforts, but also from the careful planning of the organizers: Duncan Neuhauser, William Stason, and Edward Carels. The resources to bring it about were generously provided by the Blue Shield Association. To all of them, I would like to extend my personal thanks, and the gratitude of all of the participants.

Howard S. Frazier
Director, Center for the
Analysis of Health
Practices, Harvard
Medical School

Preface

This book is addressed to the practicing physician who has become concerned about the high and rising costs of medical care. It is based on a conference held December 9 and 10, 1978, at the Harvard School of Public Health in Boston. Supported in part by the Blue Shield Association, the conference was sponsored by the Harvard School of Public Health and its Center for the Analysis of Health Practices, the Blue Shield Association, Blue Shield of Massachusetts, the American Medical Association, the American Society of Internal Medicine, the Commonwealth Institute of Medicine, and the Massachusetts Medical Society.

The importance of this topic brought together these distinguished sponsoring organizations. Although this sponsorship does not mean that the organizations like or dislike any of the ideas proposed here, it does mean that they are concerned about the costs of medical care and are urging others to be concerned, too. The opinions expressed by the authors here are their own and do not necessarily reflect those of the organizations with which they are associated, nor do they necessarily reflect the positions of the sponsoring organizations.

This book focuses on what practicing physicians can do to control these costs. Therefore, it does not consider such questions as improving hospital management, reorganizing the federal government, or reviewing options for national health insurance.

Introduction

There are three sets of organizing principles in this book based on (1) the physician's role, (2) a model for behavior change, and (3) the stages of patient-physician interaction.

THE PHYSICIAN'S ROLE

There are major variations in the volume of medical care provided to similar patients and similar patient populations. Chapters 1 and 2, in which the magnitude of the problem and practice variation are discussed, respectively, marshal this evidence. Variations in the volume of medical care are associated with large differences in costs. Physicians control a large part of the use of medical care resources, through ordering tests, prescribing medication, giving direct care, and, of course, requesting admission of patients to the hospital. Therefore, if physicians and their patients care to do so, the costs of medical care can be reduced. Dr. Steven Schroeder has empirically addressed this proposition, and Dr. Mervin Shalowitz has tackled this issue for his medical group. The reader is not expected to accept this proposition simply because it is stated. The evidence follows, however, and it is up to the reader to decide.

A MODEL FOR BEHAVIOR CHANGE

A simple model for behavior change is summarized in Figure I.1. The first prerequisite for behavior change is that physicians become aware of the costs they generate as a result of their clinical decisions. As Dr. Lawrence urges, awareness of costs can be conveyed to medical students and residents in the educational process. A number of other methods of feeding back information about costs to physicians are also proposed.

Once physicians become aware of the costs that result from what they do, they need a way of analyzing them, that is, a way of bringing costs into their decision calculus. Cost-effective clinical decision making, discussed in Chapter 8, is one technique for doing this; the costs and risks can be balanced against the benefits of clinical decisions.

Once physicians are aware of costs and have ways to analyze cost questions, they must be motivated to apply them. Behind motivation are the incentives that drive physicians' behavior. These factors include professional self-respect, peer pressure, defensive medicine resulting from the threat of a law suit, and monetary incentive, to name a few. Do incentives for physicians have to be changed?

Awareness and method (techniques) motivate direct behavior

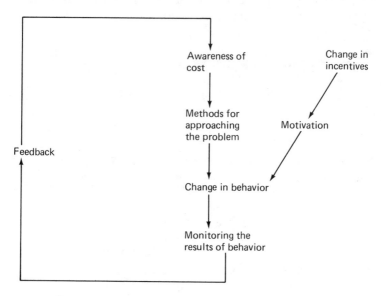

Figure I-1. Diagrammatic model for behavior change.

change. The results of subsequent behavior need to be monitored and fed back to physicians to update their awareness.

THE STATES OF PATIENT-PHYSICIAN INTERACTION

A third organizing principle relates to the sequential stages of patient-physician interaction. This interaction is shown in a simplified form in Figure I.2. The chapter numbers associated with each stage are shown in parentheses.

What leads patients to seek care? Physical and psychological conditions, culture, environment, beliefs about medical care, and personality all play important roles.

An office visit can result in various types of testing that lead to a diagnosis and a physician's decision of "no disease—no treatment," ambulatory care, or inpatient care. Inpatient care, in turn, can be subdivided into the decision to admit the patient to the hospital, a choice of diagnostic and treatment modalities, or the decision to discharge the patient. Finally, discharge can lead either to a return to the well population or to followup and extended care.

WHY BE CONCERNED WITH THE COSTS OF MEDICAL CARE?

Why be concerned about costs? Although there are many ways that this question can be approached, several ways have been selected for discussion in this book. The reader can choose which, if any, are appealing.

Physicians are one of the most highly respected occupational groups in the country. They have a high level of education and shoulder a major responsibility for the health and survival of Americans. Physicians have always been concerned with the quality of the care they provide. Why should they not also be concerned about the costs of what they do? The professional societies that sponsored this conference have, we believe, concluded that if physicians are not concerned about the costs of medical care, someone else will be. And this may well be the federal government. Thus, this provider of health care will be farther removed from understanding patients and their needs and from understanding the benefits of medical care. By being farther removed, the government will have less knowledge and, therefore, will be likely to make less intelligent decisions.

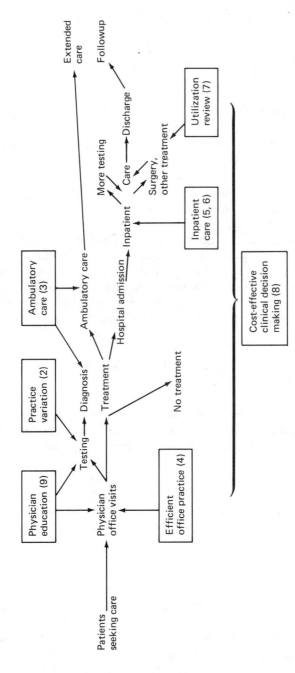

Figure I-2. Stages of the patient-physician interaction. (*Source:* Dr. Benjamin Barnes, used with permission.)

Fifty years ago physicians worried considerably about the costs of medical care because patients had to pay for their care directly. The sliding fee scale was one response to this problem, and the provision of free care to those too poor to pay for it was another. A hundred years ago, it is doubtful if a physician would recommend taking the waters at Marianbad or Hot Sulfur Springs for a month or a long trip abroad for anyone except the well-to-do. Surely, the poor could not have afforded such treatment.

Health insurance, whether it is Blue Cross-Blue Shield or insurance from private companies or the government, was created explicitly to ensure that patients could receive care without worrying about the costs. At the same time, government-funded research was specifically designed to find ways of providing better health care. Thus, yesterday's answers are today's problem, not only in the United States but also throughout the world.

The "cost crisis" has developed because physicians have been too responsive to society's desires for "first-class" medical care. Physicians have done what has been asked of them. Instead of being distressed or irritated by this turn of events, how can it be turned to the advantage? Can the issue of costs be used to introduce more precise methods of clinical decision making such as those introduced in Chapter 8? Can the issue of costs help renew our respect for ambulatory medical care and for the value of long-standing relationships between doctors and their patients? If "defensive medicine" is creating unnecessary medical costs, can a way be found to reduce the specter of malpractice suits that serves no one well except a few lawyers?

ARE THE COSTS OF MEDICAL CARE REALLY TOO HIGH?

The costs of medical care are not necessarily too high. For example, observe the behavior of the federal and state governments. On the one hand, a variety of proposals and regulations appear to be striving for cost containment; however, at the same time other governmental actions are pushing costs higher, as in the case of the stiffer requirements for safe hospital construction.

Governments express concern about the costs of the medical care for which they now pay. But if any one of the proposals for national health insurance were enacted, the federal government would pay even more for medical care. Although these examples of apparent governmental schizophrenia suggest that the costs of medical care may not be too high, after all, they should in no way lead physicians to the conclusion that they should ignore the issue of costs. Governments and consumers, alike, perceive that medical care costs are too high. Thus, it behooves physicians to analyze the costs of medical care carefully, to reduce them where possible, and to respond constructively to criticism that may be levied. Perhaps in this way the "cost crisis" can be turned into an opportunity.

PART I

The Problem

Chapter 1

Health Care Costs: The Magnitude of the Problem

*Edward J. Carels**

Our theme is that physicians must be as concerned about the cost of medical care as they have traditionally been concerned with its quality. Joe Follman, research director of the Health Insurance Association of America (HIAA), gives us a tongue-in-cheek perspective on today's health care system:

> In ancient Rome, when doctors placed total reliance in the gods, cuffing, bloodletting, and a few herbs and the fact that nature itself would eventually dispose of matters one way or another, the span of life averaged 23 years. The vast majority of the living were robust and pink cheeked and spent their meager number of years zestfully pouring, warring and whoring. Today, with modern surgical techniques, magnificent hospitals, anesthesia, miracle drugs, blood transfusions, monitoring systems, transplants and a host of other armamentaria, 46 years have been added to the Roman span of life. The majority of the living today are a cautious, wary, pallid, aching, crotchety, alcoholic, drug addicted, dieting, psychoneurotic, bilious, constipated, pill-consuming creatures who devote a considerable portion of their productive life gratefully supporting the health professions who made this delightful state of affairs possible.[1]

*Director of Research, Health Care Management Systems, Inc., La Jolla, California.

ASSUMPTIONS AND CONCLUSIONS THAT OTHERS HAVE REACHED

Health care costs literally cannot be contained. We must not kid ourselves into thinking we can or will roll back prices to the level of some less expensive previous era. It is more realistic to assume that we will slow the rate of escalation.[2] Some factors —such as inflation, population growth, and increased longevity— cannot be controlled. Together, these three factors account for more than two-thirds of the increase in costs since 1950.[3]

Physicians and hospitals are wrongly being blamed for the problem of rising health care costs and are rightfully annoyed and confused about being singled out. Who is to blame for rising costs? Everyone: hospitals, physicians, patients, labor and management, and government.[4]

To some physicians cost cutting means "Personal financial loss, increased mental and emotional stress, worried patients . . . ,

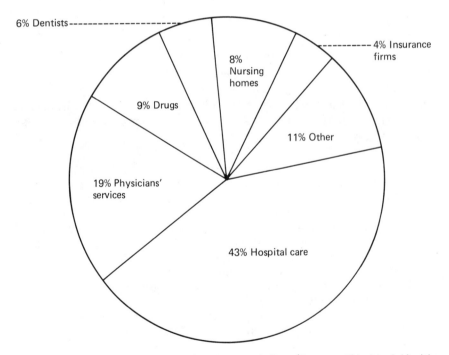

Figure 1-1. Distribution of the health care dollar. (*Source:* "National Health Expenditures, 1975," by M. Mueller and R. Gibson, *Social Security Bulletin,* 39:3-20, February 1976.)

strained relations with colleagues and lowered quality of care, along with inconvenience to many patients and real risk to a few."[5] But cutting costs need not cause any of these problems.

THE PROBLEM

Health care costs are rising faster than the overall rate of inflation—in some years they have risen twice as fast. The problem is that they show no signs of stabilization. Some fear that, left unchecked, costs will continue to spiral. Figure 1.1 indicates where the health care dollar is being spent. Note that 43 percent is going to hospitals. From Figure 1.2 we see that payments from the public are increasing more quickly than payments from other sources. To put medical care spending into perspective, consider that Americans spent more on each of the following than they spent on medical care in 1973: transportation, housing, clothing and jewelry, food, beverages, and tobacco. How were personal health care costs paid in 1976? Social Security figures indicate that, for hospital care, the government paid 55 percent,

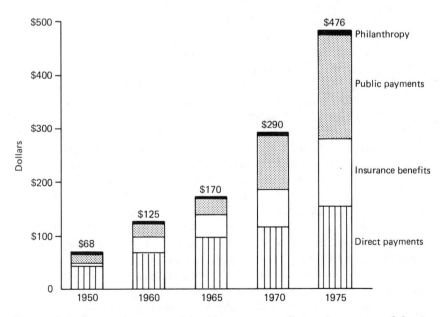

Figure 1-2. Per capita personal health care expenditures by source of funds, selected years 1950 to 1975. (*Source:* "National Health Expenditures, 1975," by M. Mueller and R. Gibson, *Social Security Bulletin* 39:3-20, February 1976.)

private health insurance 35 percent, and patients out-of-pocket 9 percent. For physicians' services, government, private insurance, and patients paid 25 percent, 35 percent, and 39 percent, respectively. Patients paid 81 percent of dentists' services and 84 percent of drug costs.[4]

Other countries are having the same problems: health care costs throughout the world are rising faster than the cost of living with or without national health insurance, and hospitals absorb the bulk of the expenditures. These trends suggest that the forces in the medical infrastructure are the same all over the industrialized world.[6] Roemer suggests that national health insurance generally increases utilization and hence spending on health services. He concludes that the United States has the weakest social insurance system of the developed countries, yet spends the most on health care; as a consequence, people get more for their money in other countries.[7]

Survey data here and in Europe indicate persistently high rates of perceived illness. Demand for health services therefore appears infinite. Consequently, a few physicians view clinical freedom as a license to ignore cost considerations altogether.[8]

CONTRIBUTING FACTORS

The number of factors contributing to rising costs are so complex and interdependent that at times they appear to defy analysis. They can be broken down into three categories.

First, the government (complicated Medicare and Medicaid regulations, which are costly to administer and can create expenses for providers; the costs of Hill-Burton construction; the fear on the part of providers of new controls, which leads some of them to rush to spend money while they still have the chance; the transfer of welfare costs to health expenditures; and the rules of Medicare reimbursement that encourage the projection of expenses to the next fiscal year are examples of reporting rules that show up as higher costs, etc.); second, factors external to the system (inflation, population slowdown, higher costs of education, increased longevity, changing lifestyles, etc.); third, factors within the system (fraud and abuse, increased specialization, new medical technology, etc.). Population growth, price increases, and increased utilization of medical care per capita combined with quality improvement have all contributed to the growth in health expenditures. Of the three factors, higher medical prices has been the most important, accounting for approximately 54 percent of the rise in costs between

1950 and 1976. Population growth and quantity and quality increases contributed 10.5 percent and 34.9 percent, respectively.[9]

To illustrate this point further, let us examine the impact on health of new medical technology alone. According to a report of the Cambridge Research Institute,[10] the following developments have occurred because of new medical technology:

1. Disease trends are changing.
2. Public expectation has been raised.
3. Doctors and hospitals are now more susceptible to medical malpractice suits.
4. Questions about priorities and ethnics are emerging.
5. Increased specialization is resulting.
6. Increased efforts at continuing medical education are now required.
7. Greater use of hospital outpatient facilities is encouraged.

Figure 1.3 illustrates the factors affecting the increases in personal health care expenditures. It depicts the rise in health care costs attributable to price increases, population growth, and changes in the system. It seems clear that the bulk of the increase in costs between

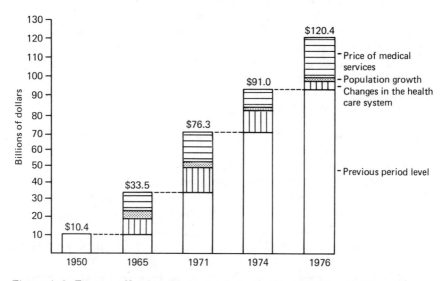

Figure 1-3. Factors affecting the increases in personal health care expenditures, selected fiscal years 1950 to 1976. (*Source:* "National Health Care Expenditures, 1976," by R. Gibson and M. Mueller, *Social Security Bulletin,* 40:3–20, April 1977.)

1974 and 1976 was caused by price increases. These facts must be considered when we deal with solutions.

As we wrestle with this problem, let us remember that some miraculous things have occurred meanwhile: American life expectancy has increased dramatically, low-income people have greater access to health care, maternal deaths have decreased, and polio has been conquered. Fluoridation appears to have halved dental decay among children at an annual cost of less than twenty cents per person. It has been estimated that the economic benefit of measles vaccine over a ten-year period exceeded $1.3 billion. The benefits in lives saved and in cases of averted mental retardation are incalculable. Medical progress seems limitless; there are now commissions to determine who is dead. In the future, we see the emergence of neonatology, recombinant DNA, and neomorphs, but on the negative side, inefficiencies exist.

INEFFICIENCIES

The issue of potential inefficiency within the health system is addressed by Dr. David Rogers: "In an effort to be 'thorough' we often seem to substitute a grueling, somewhat mindless work-up for one that is discriminating. I think we have pursued the technologic imperative to do all we are trained to do too far. . ., as our interventions have become more searching, they have also become more costly and more dangerous."[11] I would like to emphasize that most of the studies I discuss are isolated, thus raising more questions than they answer about the problem. Researchers have uncovered the following information:

1. Physicians are not aware of the costs of the services that they generate.[12]
2. Of single unit blood transfusions at a university surgical service, 34 percent were considered unnecessary.[13]
3. Antibiotics are being overused in community hospitals.[14]
4. There are inaccuracies in the reading and evaluation of lab and clinical reports used in daily practice.[15]
5. Of 1311 examined appendices, 39.6 percent were judged to be normal.[16]
6. Large percentages of persons seeking medical treatment are really suffering from emotional tension or stress-related diseases.[17,18]

7. Pertinent data are not always supplied in outpatient referrals.[19]
8. Utilization is related to defensive medicine.[20,21] Results of an AMA survey of practicing doctors show that 75 percent practice defensive medicine by ordering more tests.[22]
9. Increased utilization of diagnostic services is related to:
   a. University affiliation[23]
   b. Ownership of equipment—nonradiologists having an economic interest in equipment make greater use of x rays than other physicians[24]
   c. Age of physician and length of practice[25,26]
   d. Physician specialty[27]
   e. Wide variations in use of lab tests[28,29]
   f. Lack of correlation between frequency of lab use and either productivity or outcome[30]
   g. The fact that only 5 percent of laboratory data is actually used in treating patients[31]
   h. Lack of relationship between clinical competency and variation in laboratory costs generated by physicians[32]
   i. Wide variation in tests required upon admission by hospitals—tests tend to vary according to region and bed size[33]
10. There are large regional differences in hospital utilization[34,35] that appear to be related to the supplies of hospital beds and physicians and to surgery rates.[36,37,38] Average hospital stays were found to be longer in the Northeast than in the West.[39] Supply of general surgeons was found to be related to surgical rates at all levels of complexity.[38] Needless surgery has not been defined or quantified with any reasonable degree of accuracy.[40]
11. Physicians' decisions account for approximately 80 percent of all health care expenditures.[41]
12. Thirty-five percent of the cases treated in emergency rooms were judged unnecessary.[42] The rate of emergency utilization was six times greater for low than high economic groups.

COSTS VERSUS QUALITY

Part of the problem is a prevailing attitude in which too many people believe cost and quality are inseparable. This attitude has contributed to the rise in health care costs.

Concern about the quality of health care and its costs is not new. Hammurabi's Code, Alexander the Great, and the British plantations in Virginia (A.D. 1646) addressed fee schedules and proper utilization of drugs and services. Concern about the quality of health care began after the publication of the Flexner study of medical education in 1910. A group of surgeons who were precursors to the American College of Surgeons suggested that the quality of care should be determined by examining the results of care. These physicians, not the government or the public, took the first steps toward assuring the quality of care for the American populace.

Similarly, physicians in the Pacific Northwest created Blue Shield after the development of Blue Cross in 1929 in Dallas at Baylor University Hospital. Thus, doctors first addressed the problem of costs. As medical knowledge advanced, physicians either forgot or justifiably neglected the question of rising health care costs. Recent concern about quality assurance in organizations such as the Professional Standards Review Organization, the Health Systems Agencies, and utilization review have been stimulated by rising costs. Because of their role in medical decisions, physicians are in a unique position to help bring about a solution again.

Lewis[43] has suggested that there are three sets of cost quality curves. The first is linear and positive. He suggests that the better the quality, the higher the cost. This curve frequently describes complex and infrequent medical illnesses. The second curve is a scatter diagram, which shows no association between cost and quality. This curve describes many self-correcting illnesses. Another example is the effects of screening. Some research has failed to confirm a survivorship benefit for preventive screening.[44,45,46,47] Brooke[48] points out that if we assume that half of the 80 million people who suffer from colds annually are given optimal care for streptococcal sore throats to avoid later complications from infection, the total cost would approach $4 billion. Is this what is meant by high-quality care? Can we afford it? Most people with colds will get better without any medical care anyway.

The final curve is asymptotic. In this case, it is possible to improve care with more expenditures, although the incremental gains are negligible with increased spending. While more research needs to be done to match treatment paradigms to each curve, it seems apparent that in certain instances, we are not receiving a concomitant increase in quality for each dollar spent.

Another study suggests that changes in medical technology tend to raise rather than lower costs. Results of one study showed a steady increase in the numbers of diagnostic x rays per case (from 0.7 to

2.0) and laboratory tests per case (from 5.9 to 14.8) between 1951 and 1971.[49]

These authors[49] raise several questions:

1. Is a patient with a perforated appendix really better off when he gets almost six times as many lab tests as he did in 1951?
2. How much better off is a child with a broken forearm who has it reduced by an orthopedist instead of a general surgeon?
3. How much has increased radiotherapy improved outcomes of breast cancer?

Research has also raised other questions:

4. How much has the increased use of coronary care units improved the outcome of myocardial infarction? Additional data on CCU has shown no relationship between process and results.[50,51]
5. Is prophylactic tonsillectomy and adenoidectomy useful in relieving allergy, colds, and bronchitis? Some do not think so.[52]
6. Why do surgical claims decrease 9 percent or more after institution of second opinion programs while surgical rates generally are increasing.[53] Occasionally, treatments even cause disease in the form of adverse drug reactions.[54,55,56] Others have shown that iatrogenic diseases are directly related to length of stay.[57]

President Carter boldly asked,[58] "Can cost savings actually improve quality of care?" Perhaps they can. A pioneer program at the Blue Shield Association called "Medical Necessity" will attempt to do just that. The program will concentrate on determining the usefulness in most circumstances of certain specific procedures, leaving to the established peer and utilization review processes the examination of special cases. The areas of concentration for the program were chosen because they are difficult to identify through peer and utilization review and because they seldom represent statistical extremes. The program is aimed at discouraging payment for unproven procedures, those of dubious usefulness, redundant procedures, and those unlikely to yield additional information through repetition. According to physicians from the American College of Physicians, the American College of Radiology, and the American College of Surgeons, the following procedures appear to be of dubious current usefulness: basal metabolic rate, protein bound iodine, ballistocardiogram, phonocardiogram with interpretation and report, uterine suspension, as well as thirty-seven others. In this way doctors working with insurers have implemented powerful incentives toward not only reducing the costs of health care, but also improving the quality of care rendered to patients.

Rising costs can affect the quality of care in totally unexpected ways. To the extent that high-quality care costs more, our national ability to provide it to those who cannot pay is compromised. Rising insurance premiums have encouraged many people to reduce their scope of health care coverage. Eighty-eight percent of those leaving Blue Cross–Blue Shield mentioned cost as the primary reason for leaving.[59] It is possible that people who reduce their coverage to save money frequently forgo needed treatment because of the lack of coverage. In turn, when eventually admitted to a hospital it is likely that these people will be sicker and have a more costly episode of illness. Additional research must be carried out to detect what kind of utilization patterns such reduction of coverage causes.

Unnecessary duplication of medical technology and physician ownership of medical technology both operate to increase the cost of care and sometimes at a sacrifice of quality. When unnecessary procedures are performed, the patient is subjected to needless risk of injury or death. Fewer than 20 percent of all hospitals performing cardiac surgery perform the four to six weekly operations necessary to maintain minimum standards of quality.[58] Utilization of diagnostic x rays and laboratory tests has risen astronomically as more and more private practitioners equip their offices with technical equipment or join with colleagues in establishing profit-making laboratories.[60] Data from the federal employee health insurance program show outpatient laboratory work rose 122 percent between 1971 and 1975. During the same period outpatient diagnostic x rays increased 58.9 percent, nuclear medicine 89.7 percent, and x-ray therapy 95.2 percent.[61] Increased fees account for only a small portion of rising physician incomes. The bulk of the increase has come from increased utilization of diagnostic procedures per patient treated.[60] We must not be misled into thinking doctors are all getting rich today, however. Although physicians are the highest paid professionals now, and probably always will be, some data suggest net incomes are not really increasing much at all.[62]

MEDICINE'S IMPACT ON HEALTH

Most medical remedies attempted proceed on the assumption that more is better. More access to care as well as more medical care, insurance dollars, diagnostic screening, and so forth, are all assumed to improve health. Physicians have been trained to do everything they can for each patient. They follow the dictum, "If your mother were sick, you and I would not want it any other way."

Yet as we look at medical care in the context of the overall health of the population, one thing becomes apparent. Medical care has a very limited impact on health: it ranks fifth behind genetics, nutrition, lifestyle, and the environment.[63] Good practices in relation to smoking, weight, drinking, hours of sleep, regularity of meals, and physical activity may be more important than medical care in increasing longevity.[64] As Ann Somers indicates: "Longevity is essentially a do-it-yourself proposition. The medical care system merely patches up victims of heart attacks, automobile accidents, or attempted murder without usually affecting the underlying problems of poor diet, poor driving, or pent-up violence. A direct attack on the primary causes can only be made by efforts at prevention and education."[65] In fairness to the field of medicine, for many years the American Medical Association House of Delegates has been acting upon resolutions introduced by concerned physicians directed at diets, accidents, violence, and so on. The problem is in translating these resolutions into programs for action. One concern is financing, which is especially difficult for insurers, who are struggling to pay for the traditional forms of coverage without adding new and innovative programs. Dever clearly illustrated the impact of medical care by estimating the impact of the *health care system* (including medical care), the *environment, human biology,* and *lifestyle* on mortality. He found that lifestyle had the most significant impact on diseases of the heart, cancer, cerebrovascular disease, motor vehicle accidents, respiratory disease, and diseases of the veins, arteries, and capillaries. It is interesting to note that the federal government allocates 90.3 percent of its expenditures for the medical care system and only 1.3 percent to disease prevention.[66]

Goldbeck offers a disquieting summary: "Changing or improving health in this country will not come from expanding insurance to all citizens, not from increased technological innovations, not from increased or better distributed manpower, not by massive screening programs for all major diseases but rather from drastic changes in lifestyle."[2]

Lifestyle habits can be changed, and the public wants the help of the medical profession. Fifty-two percent of American males smoked cigarettes in 1966, and figures for 1970 showed a decrease to 42 percent. Polls show that 56 percent of the American public feels a need for more information about health and medical care. Eighty percent desired a system in which health information would be distributed by doctors and hospitals on a regular basis.[65]

SOLUTIONS

Numerous approaches to solving the problems of escalating costs have been tried over the years, and many of them were sponsored by the federal government. Government regulations have failed to accomplish much. In fact, some believe that by protecting inefficient competition, regulation hinders the introduction of cost-saving technology. There are other forces that reduce the likelihood of stopping health inflation: a projected increase in medical manpower, an increased proportion of the elderly in the population, and increases in disease prevention activities.[67] Insurers, have tried the following:

Contract limitations
Medical necessity clauses
Coordination of benefits
Coinsurance and deductibles
Benefit exclusions
Fee freezes
Second opinion

Legislators have tried:

Prospective hospital rate review
Certificate of need legislation
Professional Standards Review Organizations
Utilization review regulations
Health maintenance organizations
Rate review
Areawide health planning
Facility licensure

The characteristic that solutions attempted thus far share is that they have failed to cut costs. It seems as if there is an economic equivalent to Newton's Law: "For every action there is an equal but opposite reaction." For example, examine wage and price controls. Although PSROs and HSAs were supposed to help cut health care costs, can they be effective? Per diem rate setting can penalize efficient hospitals in which the length of time patients stay is made shorter. Certificate of need has diverted rather than checked hospital investments and has had a negligible impact upon patient costs.[68] Expanding outpatient benefits has not always produced concomitant savings in the hospital either.[69,70,71] Attempts to reduce unnecessary laboratory tests have shown that frequency of ordering tests can be curtailed.[28,29] However, reducing the number of tests ordered per patient does not cut the average laboratory cost per admission unless overall laboratory costs are reduced proportionately.[72] Hospital mergers and reductions in the physical facilities may avoid the costs of capital investment, but they help reduce operating costs only when individual departments cut expenditures for manpower and supplies.[72]

While the reasons for failure are not totally clear, two possible explanations can be advanced. First, some of the contributing factors are beyond control. Second, most of the solutions have been univariate approaches to a multivariate problem. They have failed to recognize that the factors that contribute to rising costs are not mutually exclusive but interdependent instead. The whole is equal to more than the sum of the parts, and this interrelationship of factors must be taken into consideration when working on a solution.

SOLUTION STRATEGIES

It is recommended that future solutions consider three factors. First, they should utilize cross-impact matrices.[73] Such matrices ascertain potential interactions (cross impacts) between individual factors by assigning weights and probabilities to each cause of action working through the matrix and measuring the impact that each action will have on each factor in the matrix. The use of matrices can show unexpected secondary and tertiary consequences for proposed solutions. Only in this manner will a full assessment of the effects of each "solution" be achieved.

Second, it is recommended that proposed solutions be viewed in terms of their impacts upon (1) patients, (2) physicians, (3) hospitals, and (4) the delivery system.[74]

Third, strategies should stress win/win solutions.[75] Too often compromise or inaction are the end results of problems that are difficult to solve. This has been true in health care. Physicians and hospitals want the best possible care available for each patient. On the other hand, government, insurers, employers, and patients want the highest-quality care at the most reasonable price. Both goals must be kept in mind if we are to arrive at win/win solutions. We must be prepared to accept the fact that we cannot always supply high-quality care at a reasonable price. We should concentrate our efforts on inefficiencies within the health care system, perhaps starting with diagnostic tests and surgery. By using this strategy we may develop a whole new technology—that of cost containment.

Physicians and hospitals have experimented with a number of cost-saving devices:

Use of computers to optimize admission schedules (one hospital estimates a saving of \$750,000 through such computer application)[76]

Computerized medical records and ambulatory scheduling[77]

Target rate approach for reimbursement[78]

Hospital mergers[4]

Physician assistants[79]

They have also made suggestions:

Keep a daily log of medical decisions

Write prescriptions for self-care

Print charges on order slips

Eliminate useless tests[55]

Lamb[80] provides an excellent list of suggestions for individual practitioners to consider:

Listen more to patients

Use less expensive personnel

Delegate less critical activity

Get competent secretarial help

Set up patient education centers

Enroll in practice management courses

Prescribe generics where feasible and point out attempts to save money

Buy supplies through medical cooperatives (apparently Pennsylvania has one)

Open office nights and on weekends

The conclusion reached by the Council on Wage and Price Stability was that the private sector was the best source for finding a solution. One can go further and say that physicians and hospitals must be challenged to lead the way in finding win/win solutions working with the government, insurers, and patients. They understand the problem and the system's inefficiencies better than anyone else.

There is an interdependent relationship in health care between the factors of access, quality, and cost. If we tamper with one, the others will in some way be affected. In a world with finite health care resources, a delicate balance between these factors must be struck. Apparently, for some time now the emphasis has been on access and quality at the expense of cost considerations.

CONCLUSIONS

Perhaps our best incentive for a solution is provided by former Department of Health, Education, and Welfare Assistant Secretary of Health, Dr. Charles C. Edwards, who said:

". . . the medical profession cannot reject the economic realities of the times and of the system within which they work. Failure to control costs will lead to collapse of the system. . . ."[81]

People are the source of greatness in any system. Human beings alone can produce through some degree of motivated problem solving an output greater than the sum of their inputs. I am optimistic that physicians acting without the necessity of legislation can help fulfill this prophecy.

REFERENCES

1. Follman, Joseph. Laws of Health Economics, April 26, 1971
2. Goldbeck, Willis. Major employers plunging into health benefit cost pool. *Perspective*, July 26, 1976.
3. Mueller, M. S., and Gibson, R. R. National health expenditures, fiscal year 1975. *Social Security Bull.*, 39, Feb. 1976.
4. Nelson, Harry. U.S. medical cost: We're all to blame. *Los Angeles Times*, July 18, 1977 (part of a series)
5. Orandi, A. I cut health costs and everybody suffered. *Med. Econ.*, April 4, 1977
6. Anderson, Odin W. All health care systems struggle against rising costs. *Hospitals*, 50:97-102, Oct. 1, 1976.
7. Roemer, M. I. National Health Insurance as an agent for continuing health care costs. *Bulletin of the New York Academy of Medicine*, 54:1,102-112, January 1978.
8. Owen, David. Clinical freedom and professional freedom. *The Lancet*, 1006-1009, May 8, 1976.
9. Rivlin, Alice M. Expenditures for health care: Federal programs and their effects. Congress of the United States, Congressional Budget Office, August 1977.
10. Cambridge Research Institute. *Trends Affecting the U.S. Health Care System.* DHEW Publication No. (HRA) 76-14503, Oct. 1975
11. Rogers, David E. On technologic constraint. *Arch. Intern. Med.*, 135:1393-1397, Oct. 1975.
12. Roth, Russel B. How well do you spend your patients' dollars? *Prism*, Sept. 1973, p. 16
13. Morton, John H. An evaluation of blood transfusion practices on a surgical service. *New Engl. J. Med.*, 263:1285-1287, Dec. 1960.

14. Myers, Robert S., Slee, Virgil A., and Ament, Richart P. Antibiotic study shows need for therapy audit. *Mod. Hosp.*, 100:120-124, Mar. 1963.
15. Garland, Henry L. The problem of observer error. *Bull. N.Y. Acad. Med.* 36:570-584, Sept. 1960.
16. Harding, H. E. A notable source of error in the diagnosis of appendicitis. *Brit. Med. J.*, 2:1028-1029, Oct. 20, 1962.
17. Mair, Alistair, Mair, George B., and Taylor, Andrew A. Prescription for the reduction of prescribing cost. *Brit. Med. J.*, 2:1442-1445, Nov. 12, 1960.
18. Collen, Morris F., and Garfield, Sidney R. *New Medical Care Delivery System.* NCHSR Research Project HSM 110-70-407, 1974
19. Bates, Barbara, and Torkelson, Leif O. Two methods of improving referral information: A comparative study in a university medical center. *Med. Care*, 5:418-422, Nov.-Dec. 1967.
20. American Society of Internal Medicine. *National Survey of Physicians' Office Laboratories.* U.S. Public Health Service Bureau of Quality Assurance (HSM) 110-72-341, Mar. 1975.
21. Efficacy study cites legal link. *Amer. Coll. Radiol. Bull.*, 31:7, July 1975.
22. Why most M.D.'s practice "defensive medicine." *Amer. Med. News*, Mar. 28, 1977.
23. Childs, M. A. Cholecystectomies in university and nonuniversity hospitals. *PAS Reporter* 9, Oct. 4, 1971.
24. Childs, A. W., and Hunter, E. D. Nonmedical factors influencing use of diagnostic x ray by physicians. *Med. Care* 10:323-325, July-Aug. 1972.
25. Freeborn, D. K., Baer, D., Greenlick, M., and Bailey J. Determinants of medical care utilization: Physicians' use of laboratory services. *A.J.P.H.* 62:846-853, June 1972.
26. Hardwick, D. F., Vertinsky, P., Barth, R., Mitchell, V., Bernstein, M., and Vertinsky, J. Clinical styles and motivation: A study of laboratory test use. *Med. Care* 13:397-407, May 1975.
27. Garg, M. L., Mulligan, J. L., McNamara, M. D., Shipper, J. K., and Perehk, R. R. Teaching students the relationship between quality and cost of medical care. *J. Med. Educ.* 50:1085-1091, Dec. 1975.
28. Lyle, C. B., Citron, D. S., and Sugg, R. S. Cost of medical care in a practice of internal medicine: A study in a group of seven internists. *Ann. Intern. Med.* 81:1-6, July 1974.
29. Lyle, C. B., Applegate, W. B., Citron, D. S., and Williams, O.D. Practice habits in a group of eight internists. *Ann. Intern. Med.* 84:594-601, May 1976.
30. Daniels, M., and Schroeder, S. A. Variation among physicians in use of laboratory tests: II. Relation to clinical productivity and outcomes of care. *Med. Care* 15:482-487, June 1977.
31. Dixon, R. H., and Laslo, J. Utilization of clinical chemistry services by medical house staff: An analysis. *Arch. Int. Med.* 134:1064-1067, Dec. 1974.
32. Schroeder, S. A., Schliftman, A., and Piemme, T. E. Variation among physicians in use of laboratory tests: Relation to quality of care. *Med. Care* 12:709-713, Aug. 1974.

33. Carels, E. J., and Costa I. Hospital Admission Test Survey (unpublished data). Chicago, Blue Shield Association, Aug. 1977.
34. Harris, D. M. Effect of population and health care environment on hospital utilization. *Health Serv. Res.* 10:229-243, Fall 1965.
35. Ramaswamy, K., and Tokuhata, G. C. Determinants of expenditures for physician services in Pennsylvania: Differences across counties, 1972. Paper presented at the Joint Statistical Meetings of the American Statistical Association, the Biometric Society and the Institute of Mathematical Statistics, Atlanta, Aug. 28, 1975.
36. Lewis, C. E. Variation in the incidence of surgery. *New Engl. J. Med.*, 281:880-884, Oct. 16, 1969.
37. Wennberg, J., and Gittelsohn, A. Small area variations in health care delivery. *Science*, 1102-1108, Dec. 14, 1973.
38. Wennberg, J., and Gittelsohn A. Health care delivery in Maine: Patterns of use of common surgical procedures. *J. Maine Med. Assoc.* 66:123-149, May 1975.
39. Slee, V. N. Operated patients: Regional differences in length of stay. *PAS Reporter*, 13:1-4, Dec. 1, 1975.
40. Frederick, L. How much unnecessary surgery? *Med. World News*, 17:50-60, May 3, 1976.
41. Fuchs, V. R. *Who Shall Live: Health Economics and Social Choice.* New York, Basic Books, 1974.
42. Jacobs, A. R., Gavett, J. W., and Wesringer, R. Emergency department utilization in an urban community—implications for community care. *J.A.M.A.*, 216:307-312, April 4, 1971.
43. Lewis, Charles E. The state of the art of quality assessment—1973. *Med. Care*, 12:799-806, Oct. 1974.
44. Braren, M., and Elinson, J. Relationship of a clinical examination to mortality rates. *A.J.P.H.*, 62:1501-1505, Nov. 1972.
45. Durbridge, Timothy C., Edwards, F., Edwards, R. G., and Atkinson, M. Evaluation of benefits of screening tests done immediately on admission to hospitals. *Clin. Chem.*, 22:968-971, 1976.
46. Levinson, Edwin F. An appraisal of long term results in surgical treatment of breast cancer. *J.A.M.A.*, 186:975-978, 1963.
47. Sutherland, Robert. *Cancer: The Significance of Delay.* London, Butterworth, 1960, pp. 196-202.
48. Brooke, R. H., and Davies-Avery, Allyson. Quality assurance and cost control in ambulatory care. In G. A. Giebink and N. H. White (eds.), *Ambulatory Medical Care Quality Assurance 1977.* La Jolla, Calif, La Jolla Health Science Publications, 1977.
49. Scitovsky, Anne R., and McCall, Nelda. *Changes in the Costs of Treatment of Selected Illnesses. NCHSR Research Digest Series.* DHEW Publication No. (HRA) 77-3161, July 1976.
50. Fessel, W. J., and Van Brunt, E. E. Assessing quality of care from the medical record. *N. Engl. J. Med.*, 286:134, 1972.
51. Bloom, B. S., and Peterson, O. L. End results, cost and productivity of coronary care units. *N. Engl. J. Med.*, 288:72-78, Jan 11, 1973.

52. Bolande, R. P. Ritualistic surgery—circumcision and tonsillectomy. *N. Engl. J. Med.*, 280:591–596, Mar. 13, 1969.

53. McCarthy, Eugene G., and Madelon Lubin Finkel. Second opinion elective surgery consultation program. Prepared testimony, House of Representatives, Subcommittee on Oversight and Investigations of the Committee on Interstate and Foreign Commerce, May 2, 1977.

54. Wade, Nicholas. Drug regulation: FDA replies to charges by economists and industry. *Science*, 170:775–777, 1973.

55. Barr, D. P. Hazards of modern diagnosis and therapy—the price we pay. *J.A.M.A.*, 159:1452–1456, Dec. 10, 1955.

56. McLamb, J. T., and Huntley, R. R. The hazards of hospitalization. *South. Med. J.*, 60:469–472, May 1967.

57. Schimmel, E. M. The hazards of hospitalization. *Ann. Intern. Med.*, 60:100–110, Jan. 1964.

58. Carter, Jimmy. Hospital cost containment. *Natl. J.*, 6–7, June 18, 1977.

59. Final report of research among federal employees to determine reasons for changing health benefit plans. Unpublished report, Chicago, N. W. Ayer, Aug. 9, 1976.

60. Meyer, Lawrence. Physicians and the making of money: Good pay, long hours. *Wash. Post*, 100–101, June 12, 1977.

61. *"The Buck Starts Here," Teaching Cost Awareness to Physicians.* Prepared by Professional Relations Dept., Blue Shield Association, Chicago, Sept. 1977.

62. Farber, L. Doctors' earnings: Winning the battle, losing the war. *Med. Econ.*, 176–193, Oct. 10, 1975.

63. McNerney, W. J. The quandary of quality assessment. *N. Engl. J. Med.*, 1505, Dec. 30, 1976.

64. Belloc, Nedra. Relationship of health practices and mortality. *Prevent. Med.*, 2:67–81, 1973.

65. Somers, Anne R. Public accountability and quality protection in ambulatory care. *Proceedings of Conference on Assessing Physician Performance in Ambulatory Care*, sponsored by the American Society of Internal Medicine, San Francisco, June 18–19, 1976.

66. Dever, G. E. Epidemiologic model for health policy analysis. *Soc. Indic. Res.*, 2:453–466, 1977.

67. Salkever, D. S. Will regulation control health care costs? *Bull. N.Y. Acad. Med.*, 54:1, 73–83, January 1978.

68. Salkever, D. S., and Bice, T. W. *Impact of State Certificate-of-Need Laws on Health Care Costs and Utilization.* NCHSR sponsored research, DHEW Publication No. (HRA) 106-74-57, Jan. 31, 1976.

69. Hill, D. B., and Veney, V. E. Kansas Blue Cross-Blue Shield outpatient benefits experiment. *Med. Care*, 8:143–157, March–April 1970.

70. Elniki, Richard A. Substitution of outpatient for hospital care: A cost analysis. *Inquiry*, 13:245–260, Sept. 1976.

71. Frieberg, Lewis, and Switchfield, F. E. Insurance and the demand for hospital care: An examination of the moral hazard. *Inquiry*, 13:54–60, March 1976.

72. Griffith, J. R., Hancock, W. M., and Munson, F. C. The concept of cost control in hospitals. In J. R. Griffith, W. M. Hancock, and F. C. Munson (eds.), *Cost Control in Hospitals*. Ann Arbor, Health Administration Press, 1976.

73. Gordon, Theodore J. The current methods of futures research. In Alvin Toffler, (ed.), *The Futurists*. New York, Random House, 1972.

74. McMahon, Alex. Déjà vu and health care costs controls. *Natl. J.—The Weekly on Politics and Government*, 916-917, June 11, 1977.

75. Doyle, Michael, and Straus, David. *How to Make Meetings Work*. Chicago, Playboy Press, 1976.

76. *Health Resources News*. Health Resources Administration, Department of Health, Education, and Welfare, 4, 15, September 1977.

77. Barnett, G. Octo. *Computer Stored Ambulatory Record (COSTAR)*. NCHSR funded research HS-00240, 1977.

78. Miller, Allan B. *The Solution to High Costs in Health Care Could Be Simple if Only the Facts Didn't Get in the Way*. Annual Report American Medicorp, Inc., Mar. 30, 1977.

79. Greenfield, Sheldon, Komoroff, Anthony, Pass, Theodore, Anderson, Hjalman, and Nession, Sharon. Efficiency and cost of primary care by nurses and physician assistants. *N. Engl. J. Med.*, 289, 6:305-309, Feb. 9, 1978.

80. Lamb, Robert. Health care cost containment—can we help? *Penn. Med.*, 20-25, August 1977.

81. Edwards, Charles C. Form and function in the federal health effort. *N. Engl. J. Med.*, 675, Sept. 16, 1976.

Chapter 2

Variations in Physician Practice Patterns: A Review of Medical Cost Implications

*Steven A. Schroeder**

It has almost become a cliche to assert that the physician is "the captain of the team," in Victor Fuchs's terms,[1] who controls the expenditures of medical dollars. It has been estimated that approximately 80 percent of all health care expenses are determined by physicians. Physicians decide about hospital admissions, length of hospital stay, use of hospital resources, and the site of posthospital care. They also, for the most part, determine the use of ambulatory services, such as visits to the doctor's office, laboratory and x-ray services, pharmaceutical prescriptions, and applications of medical devices. Although the figure of 80 percent is almost impossible to validate precisely (and in my opinion probably underestimates the role of consumer demand), few would quarrel with the notion that physician behavior is the single most important determinant of the costs of medical care. As such, the focus of this book—the physician and cost control—is timely and appropriate.

The purpose of this chapter is to review the extent of variation in physician practice patterns and to relate this variation to the medical cost problem. The appropriateness of examining the impact

*Associate Professor of Medicine, Health Policy Program, University of California, San Francisco.

of physician behavior on medical costs can be illustrated by the example of laboratory tests. A decision to order a laboratory test for an ambulatory or hospitalized patient is, perhaps more than any other medical service, most directly under the control of the physician. A consumer may play an active role in deciding to schedule a visit to the doctor's office, agreeing to an elective operation, referring a relative for institutionalization, or requesting medication for sleep or constipation. The more technical decision of when and how often to order laboratory tests, however, is almost exclusively the domain of the physician, particularly in the hospital setting.

Yet, if we analyze recent trends in use and expenditures for medical services, we find that costs due to laboratory tests are rising faster than any other component of medical care. In 1977 physicians ordered about 5 billion laboratory tests that cost approximately $11 billion; the annual growth in laboratory use has exceeded 14 percent since 1970.[2] The 39 percent increase in the use of lab tests for the New Mexico Medicaid population between 1971 and 1973 exceeded all other components of medical care.[3] Scitovsky estimates that expenditures for laboratory tests and x rays account for about 25 percent of all ambulatory care expenses.[4] Griner found that laboratory and x-ray tests accounted for 25 percent of the bills of hospitalized medical patients at the University of Rochester. During a five-year period at this hospital, costs attributable to lab tests increased twice as much as overall hospital costs.[5]

These recent trends to increase the use of lab tests, a physician-determined component of medical care, illustrate why it is appropriate to examine physician behavior in some detail. This chapter reviews three aspects of physician practice variations: (1) the extent to which physicians vary in the use of medical services; (2) the relation of practice variations to variables such as physician competence and outcomes of patient care; and (3) the important determinants that influence a physician's decision to order particular medical services. The chapter concludes with a brief summary of alternative strategies for medical cost containment.

PHYSICIAN VARIATION IN THE USE OF MEDICAL SERVICES

This section will discuss variation among physicians with regard to a variety of medical services, including laboratory tests and x rays, other diagnostic procedures, and hospitalization rates (including surgery). Discussions of regional variations in use of services, such as the significantly longer duration of hospital stay in the northeastern as compared to the western section of the United States, are beyond the scope of this section as is a detailed discussion of the well-known lower rates of hospital use by patients in prepaid group practices, or the substantial variations in outcomes between hospitals regardless of patient mix.[6]

The literature on differences in physician use of medical services is not large, and it is disproportionately skewed with observations from university outpatient settings and prepaid group practices. In addition, much of the literature suffers from an inability to control for case mix, thus making it difficult to know to what extent physician variation is caused by differences in the severity of illness or the demography of the patient population studied. Another methodologic problem relates to the terminology of individual lab tests. Should an SMA-12 be counted as one test or twelve? These problems of terminology tend to be more of an issue in interpreting longitudinal trends in the use of tests and are less troublesome for comparison of physician patterns at any one time. An underlying problem affecting all discussions of physician-generated medical expenses is the difficulty in separating costs from charges. Because of the paucity of data about the real costs of medical services, this discussion will focus on costs to consumers.

Variation in Lab Tests and Procedures

Most of the data on variations in physicians' use of medical services concern laboratory tests and procedures. Freeborn and colleagues at the Kaiser-Portland Health Plan showed a pattern of increasing laboratory use between 1967 and 1970, with the most increases occurring among internists. They also describe marked variations in individual patterns of lab use. Furthermore, these patterns were stable over time and did not appear to be caused by differences in case mix, although data to this effect were not presented. The authors analyzed physician characteristics in an attempt to define low users. The only significant finding was that laboratory use profiles tended to correlate with the behavior of the clinic chief ($p < .02$); utilization patterns of other physicians were low in clinics in which the chief had a low rate of laboratory use. Conversely, clinic chiefs who were high utilizers seemed to set the pattern for their clinics.[7]

Another study from Kaiser-Portland, analyzing behavior of internists and pediatricians caring for patients with upper respiratory infections, found great variation in the use of throat cultures. Individual internists cultured from 0 to 75 percent of upper respiratory infection episodes, and internists cultured the pharynx twice as often as pediatricians.[8]

Lyle and colleagues describe practice habits in a group of eight internists in Charlotte, North Carolina. Although five of eight had subspecialty interests, most of their time was spent in office-based general internal medicine. An analysis of 3475 physician-patient contacts during a three-month period showed significant variation ($p < .001$) in the volume of laboratory studies ordered among physicians. These variations held true for all aspects of laboratory work, including clinical pathology tests, x rays, and EKGs, and were not correlated with the internists' subspecialty area.[9]

Three studies of physician variation in use of lab tests were conducted by Schroeder and colleagues at the George Washington University Medical Center. One report compared charges for laboratory use (including x rays) among thirty-three faculty internists caring for a homogeneous patient population at the general medical clinic. The authors found wide variation (seventeenfold) in mean annual lab costs per patient among the physicians, as shown in Figure 2.1; the variations were not attributable to clinical characteristics of the physicians' patients. No physician characteristic studied (such as age, board certification, or medical school attended) was predictive of cost behavior. However, one specific medical practice was more characteristic of the more costly physicians: the frequency with which patients receiving diuretic therapy were tested for abnormalities of serum electrolytes. A striking difference existed among the physicians as to whether potassium alone ($4 charge) was ordered or the entire series of electrolyte determinations (sodium, potassium, chloride, and bicarbonate—$16 charge) was obtained. As shown in Table 2.1, both ratio and absolute numbers of tests were more expensive for the costly physicians.[10]

The second report from the George Washington group compared costs of lab use among twenty-one medical interns for patients hospitalized in the coronary care unit. Again, an attempt was made to control for patient mix by restricting the analysis to uncomplicated cases. Although considerable variation existed among the interns, it was less than in the previous study.[11]

The third George Washington study compared costs of lab use for ambulatory patients among thirteen faculty internists. This analysis attempted to control for case mix by examining only patients with diagnosed hypertension. Once again, variation among physicians in use of lab tests was extreme. Mean annual charges per patient

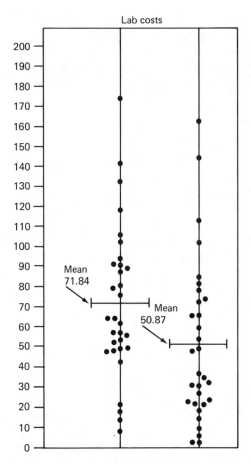

Figure 2-1. Distribution of mean annual lab costs among physicians during the two audit periods.[10] (*Source:* S. A. Schroeder, K. Kenders, J. K. Cooper et al., Use of laboratory tests and pharmaceuticals: Variation among physicians and effect of cost audit on subsequent use, *J.A.M.A.*, 225:969-973, 1973.)

ranged from $8 to $161 among the thirteen internists, with a mean of $54 and a standard deviation of $42.[12]

Studies from family practice models,[13] a general medicine clinic,[14] and a rheumatology clinic[15] have also reported significant differences among providers in their use of laboratory services.

In summary, all the reports describe great variation in the use of laboratory tests by comparable physicians, even when controlling for case mix. The variations are not obviously related to specific

Table 2.1 Frequency of K+ versus All Electrolytes for Patients Receiving Diuretics According to Physician Cost Group[10]

	Number of Determinations	
Physician Group	Potassium Only	All Electrolytes
Least costly	10	0
Middle	12	11
Most costly	17	32
Total	39	43

physician characteristics. Although most of the reports come from ambulatory settings, there is a suggestion that the variation is less extreme in hospitals.

Physician Variation in Use of Other Medical Services

Physician variation in use of medical services other than laboratory or x-ray tests is best documented in surgical services. Noteworthy are studies by Hughes and colleagues that converted all surgical operations into hernia equivalents as a means of expressing workloads. Hughes first studied nineteen general surgeons in private practice in a suburban New York community. He found that the annual number of operations varied from 47 to 569 per surgeon, with a mean of 200 and a median of 165. Annual numbers of hernia equivalents varied from 43 to 625, with means and medians of 208 and 147, respectively.[16] Hughes also found a threefold increase in the median weekly workload and more appropriate distribution of types of operations by surgeons employed in a Seattle prepaid group practice.[17] Roos and colleagues examined tonsillectomy rates in the Canadian province of Manitoba and found great variations in the frequency of performing operations and the standards of selection for operation.[18]

The study of surgical services in the United States (the "SOSSUS report") confirmed these local variations on a national basis. Table 2.2, excerpted from the condensed version of the SOSSUS report published in the *New England Journal of Medicine*, shows the distribution of operations among surgeons; Table 2.3 presents the

Table 2.2. Distribution of Physicians Who Performed Operations According to the Annual Number Performed[19]

Annual Number of Operations	% of Physicians[a]	Cumulative %
1	12.4	12.4
2–4	11.7	24.1
5–9	6.7	30.8
10–24	9.0	39.8
25–49	10.8	50.6
50–74	8.0	58.6
75–99	6.7	65.3
100–149	10.3	75.6
150–199	7.8	83.4
200–299	9.7	93.1
300–499	6.1	99.2
500+	0.9	100.1
Total	100.1[b]	

[a]Exclusive of interns and residents.
[b]2700 total.

Table 2.3. Distribution of Physicians Who Performed Operations According to Annual California Relative Values Weighted Workload[19]

Annual CRV-Weighted Workload	% of Physicians	Cumulative %
10	15.4	15.4
10–19	6.4	21.8
20–49	8.8	30.6
50–99	6.2	36.8
100–199	7.0	43.8
200–499	12.0	55.8
500–999	11.9	67.7
1,000–1,499	9.1	76.8
1,500–1,999	9.1	85.9
2,000–2,499	5.5	91.4
2,500–2,999	3.9	95.3
3,000–3,999	3.3	98.6
4,000–4,999	0.9	99.5
5,000+	0.4	99.9
Total	99.9	

same data converted to a weighted workload based on the California Relative Value Scale.[19]

It seems reasonable to assume that similar variations exist in the use of other medical services, even though documentation to that effect is minimal. For example, the report by Lyle shows statistically different rates of return appointments, use of outside consultants, and hospitalization among the eight North Carolina internists.[9] Heasman and Carstairs found great variations in median length of hospital stay for patients among different British consultants. For patients with peptic ulcer, median stay varied from six to twenty-six days; for myocardial infarction, ten to thirty-six days; for hysterectomy, three to eighteen days; and for tonsillectomy, one to five days.[20] Although comparisons between physicians yield notable variations, there tends to exist a remarkably consistent pattern when the same physician treats patients over time. This consistency is present regardless of the hospitals in which the physician practices, patient age, or disease category.[21]

Two important questions arise from these observed differences in the use of physician-controlled medical services. First, what are the benefits to patients and to society in general from varying rates of use of medical resources? Put in economic terms, what are the marginal benefits that derive from the next test, procedure, or hospital day? Second, what influences physicians to use more (or less) medical resources? In other words, what are the important determinants of physician-controlled allocation of medical resources? These two sets of questions are the focus of the next two sections.

THE RELATION BETWEEN PHYSICIAN COST BEHAVIOR AND COMPETENCE

At least four hypotheses relating physician-generated medical costs and quality of care appear possible. One hypothesis is that medical costs are positively correlated with quality of care. Thus, physicians who frequently order laboratory procedures are more thorough and conscientious, the higher costs of laboratory use being reflected in high quality of care. A second hypothesis is that medical costs are negatively correlated with quality of care. In this instance, high users would tend to be less competent physicians who attempt to compensate for clinical deficiencies by excessive reliance on tests and procedures, while low users would have greater clinical competence and could be more judicious in lab use. The third hypothesis is that medical costs are virtually unrelated to clinical competence or quality. In this case, behavior may be related to individual personality characteristics such as degree of compulsiveness or may reflect variable concern with cost effectiveness of care, but bears no relation to the quality of care delivered by the physician. The fourth hypothesis has been described by Lewis:

> One achieves a relatively high degree of quality of care (say 90 to 95% of *total* excellence) with a relatively small investment, and then the curve becomes asymptotic. It is possible in these cases to improve care with more expenditures, although the marginal gains from such continued investments may be relatively small.[22]

Unfortunately, exploration of these hypotheses is just beginning, and it is complicated by the primitive methodology available for assessing the quality of medical care. Only a handful of studies relate costs to quality. Freeborn and colleagues used internal medicine board certification as a surrogate for quality and found that board-certified physicians had lower rates of lab use than other physicians.[7] Schroeder, Schliftman, and Piemme described lab use profiles among twenty-one medical interns for uncomplicated patients in the coronary care unit of the George Washington University Medical Center. They correlated rank order of the interns according to cost profiles with their rank order according to estimated clinical competence and found essentially a zero correlation.[11]

Daniels and Schroeder compared charges from laboratory tests for ambulatory patients with hypertension among thirteen faculty internists. They correlated lab use profiles with clinical outcomes, using control of blood pressure as the dependent outcome variable. A large but not statistically significant negative correlation ($r = -.42$) existed between lab cost profiles and outcomes. This negative correlation did not seem to reflect unequal distribution of severe hypertensive patients because patients had been randomly distributed among the internists (there were no specific hypertension specialists); numbers of hypertensive complications (cerebrovascular, renal, or cardiovascular) were small and unrelated to costs or outcomes; and pretreatment blood pressure levels did not vary significantly among the internists' patients.[12]

These studies should be considered as preliminary and should highlight the need to look closely at the implications of differences in style of medical practices. It is likely that a very large number of cost benefit curves exist for individual physicians. The shape of these curves would vary according to patient variables, the particular clinical situation, and the set of determinants that influences physician behavior. It does seem clear that national concern about costs of medical care will result in increasing pressures for physicians to make explicit the marginal benefits resulting from use of costly medical resources.

DETERMINANTS OF PHYSICIANS' USE OF MEDICAL RESOURCES

As the realization grows that today's clinical practice requires physicians to make decisions about allocation of scarce medical resources, we may expect increasing efforts to analyze and quantify the elements that enter into clinical decision making. The subject of cost-effective clinical decision making has been reviewed recently.[23] This chapter will review what is known about the factors that determine physician behavior regarding the use of medical resources. For a more detailed discussion of these factors, the reader is referred to a monograph by Schroeder and Showstack prepared for the 1977 Sun Valley Forum, "The Dynamics of Medical Technology Use: Analysis and Policy Options."[24]

A list of eight important reasons and incentives for physicians to provide a particular service is presented in Table 2.4. This list omits variables such as the extent of medical insurance coverage in order to focus more directly on determinants of physician behavior. It also omits peer pressure, which is, in my opinion, a very important variable but for which no data exists, unfortunately. Available data on these eight factors are summarized below.

Perhaps the most common and important reason for a physician to perform a medical service is the belief that it will enhance the quality of care provided. Unfortunately, as has been just mentioned,

Table 2.4. Factors Influencing Physicians to Order Medical Services

1. Belief that more service will improve quality of care
2. Patient demand
3. Fear of malpractice suits ("defensive medicine")
4. Fiscal incentives
5. Medical practice variables (group vs. solo; prepayment vs. fee for service; medical specialty)
6. Educational development of the physician
7. Knowledge of costs of medical services
8. Participation in medical teaching

these is little data to document its incremental contribution to the quality of specific medical services.

A second factor is patient demand; which may influence the physician to order a particular service. Although there are no good indices by which to measure changes in patient demand over time, a dramatic increase in interest in medical events by the news media has certainly occurred. As Ingelfinger comments:

> In short, the cost of medical care may be increasing phenomenally, but the rate of its ascent is modest as compared to the steep incline of public interest in medicine, and the blast that sustains this soaring flight is supplied in large part by the activities of many news media. Comparisons of the *New York Times* Index for 1965 with that of 1975 indicates that the *Times*, in 1975, carried about four times as much medically related news as it did a decade earlier.[25]

Physicians are pressured to do things as a function of popular trends or social mores (i.e., enlarged breasts, unnecessary hysterectomy, etc.). Many patients present themselves not with medical problems, but problems in living or personality and social difficulties. According to Baumler, "people want to be pepped up, toned down, and have their natural processes interfered with . . . people have lost faith in the self-healing properties of their own bodies."[26]

The third factor is fear of malpractice suits. The practice of defensive medicine, that is, ordering services, especially procedures or tests, more with an eye on future litigation than on the patient's actual health status, has been alleged to exert an important effect on physician behavior. Few reports or empirical studies document the impetus to perform medical procedures that results from fear of possible future litigation. However, it seems obvious that many physicians may have shifted postures from "If it can help and can't hurt, do it," to "If in doubt, do it, as it may prevent a future liability suit."

There are some inferential data in this area. Jonsson and Neuhauser observe that "the volume of x-ray and laboratory tests in Swedish hospitals is about half the amount ordered for similar patients in American hospitals."[27] This is in the context of medical services provided by the state and a structured grievance redress system, with litigation as a last resort.

There are also indications that the "malpractice crisis" is changing the way in which American physicians practice. A. L. Lipson of The Rand Corporation (as reported in *American Medical News*) noted that the malpractice issue may have conflicting effects. While on the one hand, "some physicians are becoming more wary of performing 'high-risk' procedures or of dealing with patients they regard as inclined to sue, on the other hand, some physicians are performing more diagnostic tests than would otherwise be necessary."[28] Although I have seen little direct evidence about the amount of this effect, I would judge that it is in the direction of increased diagnostic tests.

A fourth incentive is monetary. Schroeder and Showstack have discussed the incentives for providing services that are created by variation in fees.[29] They presented four theoretical models of general internal medicine office practice, which are shown in Table 2.5. The four model practices consisted of fixed ratios of history and physical examination to return visits with numbers and types of medical procedures and laboratory tests increasing stepwise through the four models.

All models assumed that the specialty of the physician was internal medicine and that the "patient mix" (distribution of visits between the patients receiving a history and physical examination and a general return office visit) was constant. For purposes of their study, only patient care occurring in the physician's office was considered; patient care delivered in the hospital was omitted. The models assumed that office care accounted for approximately 85 percent of a general internist's patient care time, with the remainder being hospital care.

Models A, B, and C assumed the physician was in solo practice. Because of the larger capital investment required for equipment, Model D assumed a four-physician general internal medicine group practice. No procedures or tests were performed in the physician's office in Model A. Five basic procedures and tests were performed in Models B and C. These were an electrocardiogram, urinalysis, complete blood count (CBC), sigmoidoscopy, and tuberculin (TB) skin test. As shown in Table 2.5, the basic differences between Models B and C were the percentage of patients receiving each type of ancillary service, generally more patients in Model C receiving ancillary services than in Model B. Three additional diagnostic procedures were performed in Model D. These were a two-view chest x ray, a cardiovascular treadmill stress test, and an automated twelve-channel blood chemistry test. A Model D physician was also assumed to perform the first five procedures and tests as frequently as a Model C physician. Each model assumed that the equipment used for these services was either owned or leased by each physician or group.

Table 2.5. Percentage of Patients Undergoing In-office Procedures and Tests According to Practice Model[29]

Procedure or Test	Model A		Model B		Model C		Model D	
	H & P[a]	General[b]	H & P	General	H & P	General	H & P	General
EKG	0	0	40	7	75	10	75	10
Urinalysis	0	0	100	20	100	30	100	30
CBC	0	0	100	15	100	20	100	20
Sigmoidoscopy	0	0	25	3	50	5	50	5
TB skin test	0	0	90	3	90	5	90	5
2-view chest x ray	0	0	0	0	0	0	75	10
Stress test	0	0	0	0	0	0	20	1
SMA-12	0	0	0	0	0	0	75	10

[a] H & P = History and physical (22% of all office visits).
[b] General = General return visit (78% of all office visits).

Since this study was an attempt to illustrate incentives that are built into the reimbursement system to order ancillary services, revenue and fee assumptions were based on the system as it now operates. An attempt was made to assign fees that are commonly charged for specific services. As a proxy for a random sample of fees, a charge for each office visit and ancillary service was derived by using the relative value for that service as described in the 1974 California Relative Value Studies. This value was then multiplied by the dollar conversion factor used by the California Division of Industrial Accidents in administering the worker compensation laws during 1976 and 1977.

To account for additional physician time spent in performing and reviewing the results of procedures and tests, which would reduce total patient volume, a decrease in patient volume was built in for Models B, C, and D (5, 10, and 15 percent, respectively). Generally, it was assumed that nursing assistants and lab technicians would actually carry out most of the testing, except for performance of sigmoidoscopies and supervision of stress testing.

Income statements for each model are shown in Figure 2.2. Net income for Model A, in which no procedures or tests were done in the physician's office, was $31,000. When procedures and tests were performed in the office, and at progressively higher levels of intensity (even with a moderate *decrease* in patient volume), net income rose sharply. From the moderate case of Model B to the most technology-intensive case of Model D, there was a progressive lowering of overhead as a percentage of gross income and a progressive rise of net income. Model D, in fact, had a per physician net income almost three times that of Model A ($90,000 vs. $31,000). Net income increased from 41 percent of gross charges in Model A, to 48 percent in Models B and C, and 56 percent in Model D.

The income discrepancies illustrated by the model practices show that strong financial incentives for expensive medical care exist in our present fee-for-service pricing system. Empirical evidence that these incentives are operative in practice comes from work by Lyle and colleagues, who note that in their eight-man internal medicine practice from 40 to 48 percent of gross physician income resulted from office laboratory tests, x rays, and EKGs. If the proportion of income derived from hospitalized patients were removed, the percentage of office income from procedures would be considerably higher.[9] Although Lyle does not present data on physician time spent performing and interpreting these tests, it may be inferred from data he does present that it is proportionately less than the revenue generated.

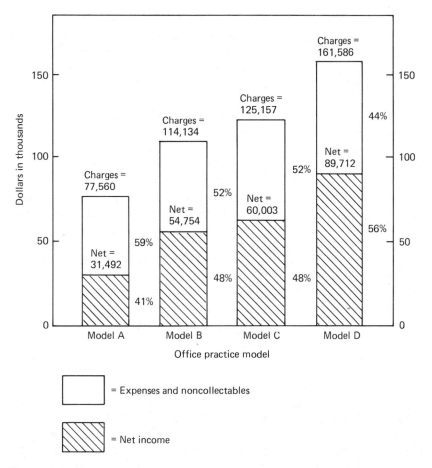

Figure 2-2. Annual gross charges, expenses, noncollectables, and net income for practice models A to D.[29] (*Source:* S. A. Schroeder and J. A. Showstack, Financial incentives to perform medical procedures and laboratory tests: Illustrative models of office practice, *Med. Care,* 16:289–298, 1978).

Thus, it appears that our current fee and pricing system provides financial incentives to perform certain medical services, particularly those involving the use of medical technology. These incentives probably have a great deal to do with the higher physician incomes generated by surgical specialists, pathologists, and radiologists.

The fifth factor influencing physician behavior is the structure and organization of the practice setting. This category includes a broad set of variables such as method of physician reimbursement, number of providers in the practice, and types of medical specialty.

Abundant evidence exists that physicians in the prepaid group practice model of health maintenance organization generate less hospital use and perhaps slightly more ambulatory and preventive services than those engaged in conventional fee-for-service practice.[30] Others support this finding that variations relate more to fiscal and organizational forms of practice than differences between physicians themselves.[31] It also appears that the use of new medical technologies such as fiberoptic gastroscopes, computerized tomography scans, and coronary bypass surgery may lag behind in the fee-for-service system.[24]

Empirical data show that physicians in fee-for-service group practices make greater use of (and resultant profit from) ancillary services such as laboratory and x-ray tests than do solo practitioners.[32,33]

A difficulty in comparing medical use across different specialties is that specialists tend to care for different types of patients with different clinical problems. Furthermore, specialists are to some extent defined by the different technologies they employ. However, some documentation of interspecialty differences does exist. Freeborn and colleagues found a greater rate of increase in laboratory use among internists compared to other specialists at the Kaiser-Portland Health Plan.[7] Garg found that patients with urinary tract infection were discharged from the hospital earlier by urologists than by internists or family practitioners and that patients of cardiologists had a shorter hospital stay than patients of family practitioners or internists when congestive heart failure, transient ischemic attack, and recent stroke were studied.[34] Another study by Garg and coworkers compared costs generated by family practitioners, internists, and cardiologists for patients with cardiovascular disease at a community hospital in the midwestern United States. Of the three specialists, internists generated the highest and cardiologists the lowest average cost per patient. These differences persisted even when controlling for case mix. It was not possible to determine whether costs of ambulatory care before or after the hospitalization were different among the specialties.[35] Although physician specialty may be a determinant of medical resource use, the data do not allow quantification of this effect.

A sixth factor that might influence behavior is the medical educational background of physicians. It has been suggested that the type of clinical exposure at both the undergraduate and graduate levels is important in shaping subsequent clinical behavior. However, data to this effect are scanty and somewhat conflicting. Pineault studied thirty-four internists practicing in the Kaiser-Permanente program in Portland. He concluded that physicians trained in medical schools and hospitals with "a scientific medical orientation" used fewer clinical and technical resources than other physicians, except under conditions of diagnostic uncertainty. He concluded that graduates of these more prestigious schools and programs are "more flexible in adjusting to the demands of the disease situation."[36] On the other hand, two studies from the George Washington University Medical Center would not explain variations in cost behavior of faculty internists by these criteria.[10,12]

Regarding general medical knowledge, physicians may practice differently because of the absence of documentation that one pattern of practice is superior to another. In other cases, there may be sufficient data available but the practicing physician may be unaware of it. Regarding training, younger physicians may be uncertain about what the chief of service wants. As a consequence, they may tend to order more tests to protect themselves from ridicule. If the physician has recently encountered several cases that were particularly difficult to solve, he or she will be more cautious and probably use more tests in treating patients with similar symptoms in the future.

Knowledge about absolute and relative costs of medical care is another factor that might influence cost behavior. For example, Schroeder and colleagues reported a 29-percent decrease in charges from laboratory use among thirty-one faculty internists after receipt of an audit describing the relative cost behavior of the internists for a set of comparable ambulatory patients. Cost reduction was significantly greater ($p < .01$) for physicians ranked in the most costly third of the audit.[10] El-Khatib and colleagues compared hospital charges of two groups of medical residents, one of which was exposed to an educational program about charges for common diagnostic tests. Charges for ancillary tests and procedures were 25 percent lower in the experimental group, although length of hospital stay and room charges were similar.[37] A simulated clinical decision-making program based on computer-stored information produced similar results.[38] That physicians and medical students tend to be unaware of charges for diagnostic tests has been well documented.[39,40,41] These findings suggest that educating physicians about medical costs may be a strategy to consider in implementing cost containment programs.

The eighth factor listed in Table 2.4 is participation in medical teaching. The extent to which practicing in an educational setting influences the costs of medical care seems answerable by two straightforward accounting processes. First, what proportion of the hospital budget is attributable to salaries for the house staff and to teaching activities of the clinical faculty? And second, to what extent does the teaching process alter the process of care such as increasing the length of stay or increasing the use of consultative and diagnostic services such as laboratory and x-ray tests? However, the question is made a great deal more difficult by the problem of case mix. That is, most university hospitals care for an unusually large percentage of patients with relatively complicated illnesses or provide special services such as renal transplantation.

The inability to control effectively for case mix has flawed most attempts to measure hospital teaching costs. However, some interesting work has been done. Griner found specific patterns of lab overuse at the Strong Memorial Hospital in Rochester, New York, including CBCs, serum electrolytes (which for some patients in intensive care were performed four or more times per day), BUNs, chest x rays and sputum cultures as routine daily procedures in the pulmonary intensive care unit, and routine SGOT determinations.[5]

In a followup study, Griner compared expenditures for patients with acute pulmonary edema before and after the opening of an intensive care unit. Although the mortality rates did not change, duration of hospitalization increased by 2.3 days and expenditures by 50 percent. Particularly striking were increases in lab tests, especially arterial blood gases, which showed a sevenfold increase in frequency coincident with the opening of the intensive care unit.[42]

Dixon and Laszlo analyzed laboratory tests for patients on the medical service of the Durham VA Hospital. They judged the usefulness of each test on the basis of four criteria: (1) Did it generate an order for medication or the need for other care? (2) Were the results considered in planning for subsequent patient care? (3) If abnormal, was the test repeated appropriately? (4) If normal, was it evident that the test ruled out diagnostic considerations? Analysis of lab tests on fifty randomly selected patients showed that only 5 percent of tests yielded a positive answer to any of these criteria. When the house staff was limited arbitrarily to eight lab tests per patient per day, the percentage of appropriate tests increased to 23 percent.[43]

Schroeder and O'Leary compared the experience of 450 hospitalized patients of thirteen faculty internists at two hospitals—one a major university medical center and the other a nearby community hospital. After controlling for type and severity of illness, they found that duration of hospital stay was equivalent at the two hospitals but that frequency of consultations, lab tests, and radiological procedures was significantly higher at the university hospital. Of the

54 types of diagnostic tests and procedures ordered for these patients, 21 were performed significantly more often at one hospital, with 19 of the 21 ordered more frequently at the university hospital; virtually all of these 19 tests were blood tests. The increased frequency of testing at the university hospital accounted for 56 percent of the differences in charges between the two hospitals.[44] Thus it appears that the teaching setting is associated with increased laboratory use, possibly to an excessive degree.

Personal attributes of the physician can also influence practice variations. These factors include age, specialty, board certification, interest in continuing medical education, and personality factors. Pineault suggests that under conditions of uncertainty in which the diagnosis is unknown, physicians tend to use more services.[45] Physicians may utilize testing to impress peers or simply to acquire more knowledge about the patient's case. Different physicians with access to the same data about patient care may use the data differently because of alternative problem-solving techniques and styles and they may arrive at different conclusions.

Practice variations can also influence medical care usage. Availability and access to new diagnostic technology may influence practice patterns. If machinery or equipment is available, the doctors will generally use it; location of practice can indirectly relate to this. A practice near a laboratory or hospital is more likely to make greater use of these facilities than a practice for which they are not so accessible. Another relevant practice variable is that of work load. The types of patients or the number of patients (i.e., patient load) that the physician has will undoubtedly affect the way in which ancillary testing is utilized. In short, time pressures will create variations in and of themselves.

This section has summarized available evidence about the impact of eight different factors on the behavior of physicians with regard to the use of medical resources. Table 2.6 contains a summary of this section according to my subjective estimates of the evidence, with each factor scored on a scale from 1 to 4+.

CAN PHYSICIAN BEHAVIOR
BE CHANGED?

It is assumed that physician behavior in the use of medical resources is susceptible to change. Some data are available to support this assumption. Three recent studies document a decrease in utilization of medical resources after institution of state or provincial

Table 2.6. Summary of Evidence Regarding Factors Influencing Physician Behavior in Use of Clinical Resources

Factor	Summary of Evidence
1. Improve quality	±
2. Patient demand	++
3. Fear of malpractice suits	++
4. Fiscal incentives	++++
5. Practice variables	
Group vs. solo	++
Specialty	+
Prepayment vs. fee for service	++++
6. Educational background	±
7. Knowledge of medical costs	++
8. Medical teaching	+++

surveillance programs associated with feedback of the information to physicians. Tonsillectomy rates in Vermont declined 46 percent in four years after feedback of data showing regional variations in this operation. In the Vermont area with the highest operation rate, physicians reviewed the indications for tonsillectomy and adopted a second-opinion procedure for surgical candidates. This area showed an 89-percent decline in numbers of tonsillectomies.[46]

In 1970, the College of Physicians and Surgeons in the province of Saskatchewan appointed a committee to investigate rapid rises in the provincial hysterectomy rate. The committee compiled a list of indications for this procedure and classified hysterectomies as either justified or unjustified. The total number of hysterectomies dropped by 33 percent subsequent to the review process, and the proportion of unjustified hysterectomies decreased from 24 percent at the time of the first review to 8 percent.[47]

A peer review system reviewing the usage and appropriateness of antibiotics in New Mexico Medicaid recipients was coupled with programs to educate the physician population and to deny payment for inappropriate use of antibiotics. This system resulted in more appropriate antibiotic use and reduced the use of injections by 60 percent.[3]

Studies from smaller group settings show conflicting results. Freeborn documented that physician lab use declines with length of employment at the Portland Kaiser program and that the lab use profiles of the clinic chief set the pattern for other physicians.[7]

Schroeder demonstrated a 29-percent decrease in lab use charges among faculty internists after a feedback audit in the medical out-patient department.[10] The study by El-Khatib showed that an educational program in medical costs led to a 25-percent decrease in lab charges by medical residents.[37] Eisenberg evaluated the effectiveness of an educational program in decreasing use of prothrombin time determination by house staff physicians at the Philadelphia VA Hospital. Six months after the educational program, use of this test routinely on admission had decreased significantly from 87 percent to 55 percent. However, twelve months later the use of the test had returned to its initial levels.[48] On the other hand, Eisenberg at the hospital of the University of Pennsylvania[49] and Marton at the Palo Alto VA Hospital[50] were not able to change laboratory use patterns of medical house officers by feedback audit systems concentrating on appropriate use of laboratory tests. One explanation of the failure of the latter two studies is that patterns of laboratory use by house officers are so strongly reinforced by existing incentives that voluntary programs initiated by chief or senior residents will be ineffective.

On balance, although it does appear that physician behavior is susceptible to modification, little is known about either the impact or side effects of the various strategies to change this behavior. Just as the factors that influence physician behavior are complex and poorly understood, attempts at modifying physician behavior must take into account the broad system variables, such as those listed in Table 2.6, as well as the unique factors operating in specific practice settings. The documented importance of understanding and modifying physician cost behavior in this time of accelerating medical costs strongly suggests a need for more research support from those with a stake in cost control, specifically the U.S. government, other third-party payers such as Blue Shield, and other concerned parties including medical and hospital associations, labor, and management.

STRATEGY CONSIDERATIONS FOR PRACTICE VARIATIONS

The first strategy is to identify variations. Only by identifying the problem (such as making variations visible) can we expect to find solutions. The contribution of each factor to the overall problem of variations must be determined before any changes can be expected to occur. We should look for variations and focus our efforts in quality assurance and cost containment upon these areas. Once documented, practice variations should be presented to the medical community in the hopes of changing behavior. The elimination of unnecessary radiology exams and careful analysis of all hospital departmental spending have been effective in restraining costs in one hospital.[51] Second, we must qualify our efforts to acknowledge that variations may not necessarily all be considered problems. Different practice styles may provide good outcomes nevertheless. Third, sizable variations suggest that the greater the variation the less the certainty about the problem in question. In that sense, variations may act as a measure for review by quality assurance programs. High variations may indicate to quality assurance personnel that the optimal approach to the diagnosis and treatment of a particular illness is unknown. In turn this should stimulate more careful research and wider dissemination of research results. Fourth, physician personal security is an underlying motivation of many of the factors contributing to increased usage of medical care services. Currently, physicians have little incentive to hold down medical service utilization unless incentives such as capitation, prepayment, or an other alternative can be developed and widely implemented. Thus, most cost containment strategies applied to fee-for-service practices will be hampered.

Fifth, criteria development and standard setting in medical treatment tend to be encyclopedic and therefore raise rather than lower costs. If physicians adhered to most treatment standards and criteria that have already been set by expert committees, there would be significant increases in the costs of medical care. Sixth, we must clarify the role played by each factor in affecting physician utilization of services. Determinations should be made about the degree to which these have an impact on medical care costs. Once the causes for variations and increased medical care utilization are defined and their contribution to unnecessary medical care costs are evaluated, strategies for cost containment should be devised for each factor. Different strategies will be appropriate for each factor. For some factors, such as physician lack of awareness of a cost-effective practice, education may be the best solution. For others, such as fiscal incentives, changes in reimbursement and institutional structure will have to be made. Seventh, the processes used to measure variation in physician practices must be accurately recorded and improved, since these have been shown to affect the magnitude of variations.[52]

CONCLUSION

Given the importance of physician behavior in the use of medical resources and our increasing national concern about the costs of medical care, what actions ought we to consider? The most obvious conclusion from this chapter is that we need to know more about how physicians behave, how their behavior might be changed, and what consequences would result from such changes.

Unfortunately, because of the current political urgency about cost control and the likely complexity of research into physician behavior, we will probably hear calls for action before we understand the issue fully. Indeed, such action plans have been widely discussed in the medical, lay, and political press during the past decade. In the light of what we currently know about physician behavior, what strategies seem most applicable at this time?

The first area to consider is that of physician supply. Like hospitals, physicians seldom sit idle. Ginzberg estimates that the net addition of one physician adds approximately $250,000 to the annual operating cost of the health care enterprise, most of it due to technology use.[53] It is also likely that specialists, who tend to be defined clinically by specific and costly technology use, generate more costs than generalists. As Reinhardt has noted, physicians have the capacity to generate sufficient demand so as to meet targeted income levels.[54] Clearly then, adjusting the number and type of physicians produced would be an important and effective step in medical cost control. However, this move would not be popular politically and might adversely affect the access to care in underserved areas. Furthermore, the long lag time required to physician training limits this strategy to a long-range solution.

Another strategy is to alter the fiscal incentives created by our current fee-for-service reimbursement system. If these built-in incentives are not changed, and if one assumes that the individual physician will continue to be able to allocate medical resources based on his or her judgment, then it seems less likely that any other cost containment mechanism will be successful.

Other strategies short of these two fundamental reforms are likely to be less controversial as well as less successful. Encouraging the growth of prepaid group practices continues to be an important approach to cost control, as does educating the public and physicians about the nature and extent of medical costs. Second-opinion programs for elective surgery have resulted in decreased frequency of these operations.[55] While I agree with the experience of Orandi[56] that voluntary cost control by itself is apt to be an ineffective and unpopular action, it seems important that we begin to discuss issues of medical costs broadly, both within the medical profession and for the general public. For the issue of cost control is really a social issue that is dependent on a broad political consensus. Rational decisions about the appropriate level of medical expenditures will, in my opinion, not be possible without a political consensus concerning medical resource allocation.

The following suggestions have been made to influence practice variations and reduce costs:

1. Create incentives for medical education in cost containment. One approach might be to offer continuing education credits for attending courses in cost effectiveness. Another would be to institute medical school courses in socioeconomics as a part of the mandatory curriculum.
2. Publish costs associated with case studies such as those from the Massachusetts General Hospital that are reported in the *New England Journal of Medicine*. At the end of each case study the total cost of the treatment could be presented, hopefully pointing out the cost rationale for the diagnostic and treatment regimen.[57] Practicing physicians must be convinced that costs are a legitimate concern to model teaching facilities, and hopefully this example will be emulated.
3. Review current procedural terminology (CPT) for areas that encourage increased utilization or billing of services.
4. Put services on a capitation or prepaid basis. This could be confined only to lab tests and x rays or extended throughout the entire range of health care services rendered.
5. Encourage insurers to charge physicians for ordering tests unnecessarily.
6. Improve the quality of laboratory testing to minimize the number of false positives that must subsequently be retested. It should be realized that the high volume of tests ordered is contributing greatly to this decreased quality of laboratory testing.
7. Review a physician's style of practice in treating a given patient problem and determine the reasons why this physician does things in selected ways.
8. Place a ceiling on what physicians can spend for certain things such as ancillary services. In short, put physicians on a budget.

This, in turn, would force physicians to decide what is necessary and what is not.

9. Create positive incentives for using fewer ancillary tests. This could be accomplished by permitting doctors to share in any savings or participate in certain bonus schemes that might accrue from the prudent use of selected services.

10. Create a cost containment journal or newsletter for physicians to exchange ideas and research relating to cost containment in both ambulatory and institutional practice settings.

11. Provide physicians and patients alike with copies of hospital bills. Although there is guarded optimism about this point, it is generally agreed that both the giver and receiver of health care services must be sensitive to the economic impact of the treatment transaction.

REFERENCES

1. Fuchs, V. R. *Who Shall Live: Health Economics and Social Choice.* New York, Baisc Books, 1974.
2. Fineberg, H. V. Clinical chemistries: The high cost of low-cost diagnostic tests. In S. Altman and R. Blendon (eds.), *Medical Technologies: The Culprit Behind Health Care Costs?* DHEW, Sept. 1979.
3. Brook, R. H., and Williams, K. N. Evaluation of the New Mexico peer review 1971-1973. *Med. Care,* 14:1-122, Supplement, 1976.
4. Scitovsky, A. A. Changes in treatment and the costs of "common" illness. In S. Altman and R. Blendon (eds.), *Medical Technologies: The Culprit Behind Health Care Costs?* DHEW, Sept. 1979.
5. Griner, P. F., and Liptzin, B. Use of the laboratory in a teaching hospital: The implications for patient care, education, and hospital costs. *Ann. Intern. Med.,* 75:157-163, 1971.
6. Staff, Stanford Center for Health Care Research. Comparison of hospitals with regard to outcomes of surgery. *Health Services Research* 11, 2:112-127, Summer 1976.
7. Freeborn, D. J., Baer, D., and Greenlick, M. R. Determinants of medical care utilization: Physicians' use of laboratoıy services. *Am. J. Public Health,* 62:846-853, 1972.
8. Bristow, J. D., Hurtado, A. V., Greenlick, M. R., et al. A study on ambulatory medicine—Patterns of care and outcomes in upper respiratory infection. Unpublished data.
9. Lyle, C. B., Applegate, W. B., Citron, D. S., et al. Practice habits in a group of eight internists. *Ann. Intern. Med.,* 84:594-601, 1976.
10. Schroeder, S. A., Kenders, K., Cooper, J. K., et al. Use of laboratory tests

and pharmaceuticals: Variation among physicians and effect of cost audit on subsequent use. *J.A.M.A.*, 225:969-973, 1973.

11. Schroeder, S. A., Schliftman, A., and Piemme, T. E. Variation among physicians in use of laboratory tests: Relation to quality of care. *Med. Care*, 12:709-713, 1974.

12. Daniels, M., and Schroeder, S. A. Variation among physicians in use of laboratory tests: II. Relation to clinical productivity and outcomes of care. *Med. Care*, 15:482-487, 1977.

13. Wright, D. D., Kane, R. L., Snell, G. F., et al. Costs and outcomes for different primary care providers. *J.A.M.A.*, 238:46-50, 1977.

14. Charles, J. G., Stimson, D. H., and Rogerson, C. L. Analysis of a group practice: Preliminary findings from a problem oriented information system. Working paper no. 9, San Francisco Veterans Administration Hospital, 1977.

15. Bombardier, C., and Fries, J. F. Variations in the costs of illness: A pilot study with rheumatoid arthritis. Unpublished data.

16. Hughes, E. F. X., Fuchs, V. R., Jacoby, J. E., et al. Surgical workloads in a community practice. *Surgery*, 71:315-327, 1972.

17. Hughes, E. F. X., Lewit, E. M., Watkins, R. N., et al. Utilization of surgical manpower in a prepaid group practice. *N. Engl. J. Med.*, 291:759-763, 1974.

18. Roos, N. P., Roos, L. L., and Henteleff, P. D. Elective surgical rates—do high rates mean lower standards? *N. Engl. J. Med.*, 297:360-365, 1977.

19. Nickerson, R. J., Colton, T., Peterson, O. L., et al. Doctors who perform operations: A study on inhospital surgery in four diverse geographic areas. *N. Engl. J. Med.*, 295:921-926, 982-989, 1976.

20. Heasman, M. A., and Carstairs, V. Inpatient management: variations in some aspects of practice in Scotland, *Brit. Med. J.*, 1:495, 1971.

21. Praiss, I. A study of the variations in the use of hospital services within the practices of individual physicians. Thesis. The Johns Hopkins University, June 1971.

22. Lewis, C. E. The state of the art of quality assessment—1973. *Med. Care*, 12:799-806, 1974.

23. Weinstein, M. C., and Stason, W. B. Foundations of cost effectiveness analysis for health and medical practices. *N. Engl. J. Med.*, 296:716-721, 1977.

24. Schroeder, S. A., and Showstack, J. A. The dynamics of medical technology use: Analysis and policy options. In S. Altman and R. Blendon, eds., "Medical Technologies: The Culprit Behind Health Care Costs?" Washington, D.C., Department of Health, Education, and Welfare, Sept. 1979.

25. Ingelfinger, F. J. Shattuck lecture—The general medical journal: For readers or repositories? *N. Engl. J. Med.*, 296:1258-1264, 1977.

26. Baumler, Robert A. The problem isn't doctor supply—it's patient demand. *Med. Econ.*, Sept. 13, 1971, pp. 313-317.

27. Jonsson, E., and Neuhauser, D. Medical malpractice in Sweden. *N. Engl. J. Med.*, 294:1276-1277, 1977.

28. Study shows liability crisis effects. *Am. Med. News*, Mar. 7, 1977, p. 1.

29. Schroeder, S. A., and Showstack, J. A. Financial incentives to perform medical procedures and laboratory tests: Illustrative models of office practice. *Med. Care*, 16:289-298, 1978.

30. Roemer, M. I., and Shonick, W. HMO performance: The recent evidence. *Milbank Mem. Fund Q.*, 271-317, Summer 1973.
31. Eisenberg, J. M., Whitney, A. M., Kahn, L. T., et al. Patterns of pediatric practice by the same physicians in a prepaid and fee-for-service setting. *Clin. Res.*, 20, 4:736, 1972.
32. Bailey, R. Economies of scale in medical practice. In H. Klarmein (ed.), *Empirical Studies in Health*. Baltimore, Johns Hopkins Press, 1970, pp. 255-277.
33. Ernst, R. Ancillary production and the size of physician's practice. *Inquiry*, 13:371-381, 1976.
34. Garg, M. L., Mulligan, J. L., Glibe, W. A., et al. Physician specialty: Quality and cost of inpatient care. Paper presented at the annual meeting of the American Public Health Association, Washington, D.C., November 1977.
35. Garg, M. L., Mulligan, J. L., MacNamara, M. J., et al. Teaching students the relationship between quality and costs of medical care. *J. Med. Educ.*, 50:1085-1091, 1975.
36. Pineault, R. The effect of medical training factors on a physician's utilization behavior. *Med. Care*, 15:51-67, 1977.
37. El-Khatib, M., Skipper, J. K., Glibe, W., et al. Physician's knowledge of costs: Effects on utilization behavior. Abstract submitted to the American Public Health Association annual meeting, Washington, D.C., 1977.
38. Freeman, R. A. Cost containment (letter to the editor). *J. Med. Educ.*, 51:157-158, 1976.
39. Skipper, J. K., Smith, G., Mulligan, J. S., et al. Medical students' unfamiliarity with the costs of diagnostic tests. *J. Med. Educ.*, 50:683-684, 1975.
40. Skipper, J. K., Smith, G., Mulligan, J. L., et al. Physicians' knowledge of costs: The case of diagnostic tests. *Inquiry*, 13:194-198, 1976.
41. Roth, R. B. How well do you spend your patient's dollars? *Prism*, September 1973, pp. 16-17.
42. Griner, P. Treatment of acute pulmonary edema: Conventional or intensive care? *Ann. Intern. Med.*, 77:501-506, 1972.
43. Dixon, R. H., and Laszlo, J. Utilization of clinical chemistry services by medical housestaff. *Arch. Intern. Med.*, 134:1064-1067, 1974.
44. Schroeder, S. A., and O'Leary, D. S. Differences in lab use and length of stay between university and community hospitals. *J. Med. Educ.*, 52:418-420, 1977.
45. Pineault, R. The effect of prepaid group practice on physicians utilization behavior. *Med. Care*, 14, 2:121-136, Feb. 1976.
46. Wennberg, J. E., Blowers, L., Parker, R., et al. Changes in tonsillectomy rates associated with feedback and review. *Pediatrics*, 59:821-826, 1977.
47. Dyck, F. J., Murphy, F. A., Murphy, J. K., et al. Effect of surveillance on the number of hysterectomies in the province of Saskatchewan. *N. Engl. J. Med.*, 296:1325-1328, 1977.
48. Eisenberg, J. An educational program to modify laboratory use by House Staff. *J. Med. Educ.*, 52:578-581, 1977.
49. Eisenberg, J., Garner, L., Williams, S., et al. Computer based chart audit to detect over-utilization of laboratory tests. *Med. Care*, in press.

50. Marton, K. I. Factors associated with utilization of the laboratory. Abstract submitted to The Robert Wood Johnson Clinical Scholars Program Annual Meeting, Chicago, 1977.
51. Macewan, D. W., and Kiernan, M. K. Methods of radiology cost restraint in a teaching hospital. *J. Can. Assoc. Radiol.*, 24:188-191, June 1973.
52. Kessner, D. M. Quality assessment and assurance: Early signs of cognitive dissonance. *N. Engl. J. Med.*, 298:7, 381-386, Feb. 16, 1978.
53. Ginzberg, E. Paradoxes and trends: An economist looks at health care. *N. Engl. J. Med.*, 296:814-816, 1977.
54. Reinhardt, U. *Physician Productivity and the Demand for Health Manpower.* Cambridge, Mass., Ballinger, 1975.
55. McCarthy, E. G., and Widower, G. W. Effects of screening by consultants on recommended elective surgical procedures. *N. Engl. J. Med.*, 291:1331-1334, 1977.
56. Orandi, A. I cut health care costs and everybody suffered. *Med. Econ.*, April 1977, pp. 209-222.
57. Schroeder, S. A. Costs in the case records (letter to the editor). *N. Engl. J. Med.*, 298:464, 1978.

PART II

Ambulatory Care

Chapter 3

Cost Containment and
Ambulatory Medicine

Warren M. Kleinberg*

For a complete discussion of the present and future role of ambulatory health services in the containment of health care costs, all sectors in which the responsibility for cost lies—professional, institutional, governmental, and societal—must be considered.

Furthermore, a number of specific questions must be raised and addressed, such as:

1. Can increased emphasis on ambulatory health services save money?
2. Can ambulatory services offer reasonable alternatives to hospitalization? If so, under what circumstances? For what diseases?
3. What are the advantages and disadvantages of different ambulatory practice alternatives?
4. What has been the effect of our past and current regulatory and reimbursement policies on the delivery of ambulatory health services?
5. Can education for ambulatory medicine make a difference?

Over the past twenty-five years, expanding health services and increasing public expectations have produced a health care cost

*Department of Clinical Medicine, Medical College of Ohio.

spiral. Through Medicaid and Medicare, the government has been brought directly into providing reimbursement for health services and, hence, into attempts to control costs, particularly in hospitals. Professional standards review organizations were an outgrowth of governmental concern over costs, and the prospect of a national health insurance program has fueled this concern. The dramatic increases in health care costs have resulted from several sources: the inflation of medical prices, increased utilization of services, and technological developments.[1] As an example, the struggle to be up to date with medical technology has fostered much unnecessary duplication of expensive technology in hospitals, thereby driving up per-diem room rates. Increases in the numbers of physicians have also contributed to the problem. In the past ten years there has been a 50 percent increase in the number of medical students[2], and by 1980, there will be twice as many medical students graduating as there were in 1964. In the absence of a competitive market for medical services, each physician is estimated to increase the cost of medical services by $300,000.[3]

Ambulatory services may provide an alternative to hospital care. In selected studies, it has been shown that when the population and numbers of physicians were stable, expansion of ambulatory services led to a substantial reduction in the utilization of emergency rooms and hospital beds.[4,5,6,7] In other studies, however, expanded ambulatory services have added to the total cost of care.[8,9]

If ambulatory health services do create an alternative to hospitalization, the impact of these services on hospital systems has to be considered.[10] In Toledo, Ohio, for instance, there is a surplus of hospital beds. The increasing number of ambulatory services, as well as the competition among the hospitals themselves, has created a situation where, to solve the problem of health care costs and services, it would mean closing one of the hospitals.[11] The prospect of closing a hospital is not pleasant to the hospital administrator, to the physicians who use the hospital, or to the community that has learned to depend on it.

Within ambulatory services, practice variations are numerous; community health needs vary and practice pressures differ both within a community and between differing communities.[12] Medical practice in the inner-city ghetto, for example, is different from that in a rural or a suburban community.[13] Differences in patient flow mechanisms, utilization patterns, and transportation problems all exist.[14] In addition, some communities have trouble attracting adequate numbers of physicians. Medicine, like many other free enterprise systems, goes where the money is.[3]

Time and motion studies in private practices, group practices, and clinics, by revealing inefficiencies, have helped to create better scheduling systems and better utilization of personnel and equipment.[15,16] Such systems evaluations have been helpful in showing physicians where their patients come from and where physicians' time is spent.[17]

Contributing to health inflation have been the open-ended policies of the third-party payers and the federal government.[9,18] Incentives to hospitalize patients and reluctance to expand ambulatory care coverage under existing risk formulas have fostered hospital care over the alternative of ambulatory services. Despite this, however, physician office visits per patient per year has doubled in the past twenty years.[2,9]

If hospital utilization is not decreased, further expansion in ambulatory service will only escalate health care costs.[19] Congress is currently disinclined to pass a national health insurance bill because of previous experience with the open-ended nature of Medicare and Medicaid and the near bankruptcy of the welfare and Medicaid systems in some states.[20,21]

Fuchs and others have noted that the way in which physicians are taught in medical school and residency programs strongly influences their subsequent practice decisions.[8,22] Because physicians are trained to depend on hospitals and on technological services that are not available readily to them in the office, the trend toward hospital care is accentuated. A study done at Indiana University is a case in point.[23] During their first two years in practice, physicians referred to the local specialty clinic many innocent heart murmurs in children and a wide variety of chest pains in adults. In subsequent years of practice, the nonpathological referrals dropped by almost 75 percent without any evidence of underdiagnosis. The logical conclusion is that it took two years to unlearn the behaviors developed during residency training.

Several components of ambulatory care have been proposed as special targets for decreasing the cost of medical care. They include periodic health examinations and multiphasic screening, patient education, self-care, home care programs, the use of other health professionals, and ambulatory surgery. The following sections will focus, in turn, on each of these components.

SCREENING

The routine physical examination has been proposed as a means of preventing health problems and detecting diseases before they become clinically evident.[24] Experience with such screening programs, however, has not shown much impact upon the overall health, morbidity, or mortality of selected populations,[25] and most studies that have indicated positive effects have been poorly controlled.[26,27]

It has been estimated that health expenditures would increase by $10 to $15 billion a year if every individual in the United States were to receive the currently recommended frequency of health examinations.[7] Unless it can be shown that these examinations reduce the costs of subsequent hospitalizations or severe illness, insurance companies will be reluctant to underwrite their costs. It remains to be demonstrated that a preventive health-oriented system produces better results than a complaint-oriented system.[1] In fact, a past president of the American Medical Association boasted that he had not had a checkup in twenty years and that no one could prove to him that he was any worse off as a result.[28]

Multiphasic screening is a variation of the routine periodic health examination that combines several separate screening tests into a single program. Its goals are to detect selected disease processes in their latent or early symptomatic stages, to identify persons at increased risk of disease, and to serve as a triage mechanism for medical care delivery. Screening procedures that are frequently included are chest x rays, pulmonary function studies, blood chemistry and hematology, body development assessment, vision tests, tonometry, hearing tests, urine tests, cytology, electrocardiography, blood pressure examinations, and rectal examinations.[25,26,27,29]

At the present time there is no clear-cut evidence that presymptomatic detection and treatment through multiphasic screening prevents progression of most of the diseases being screened for or that it reduces the subsequent need for prolonged and costly treatments.[1,30] Nor is there any evidence that multiphasic screening reduces morbidity and disability or extends the life span of the participants. One of the consequences of a major increase in multiphasic screening would be an increased need for followup facilities and health manpower.[25] The short-term costs incurred would be a difficult burden for the underwriters of the cost of health care.[8]

Another problem is that the patient populations reached by multiphasic screening programs, often, are not those that might benefit most from them. The hard-core poverty groups with high prevalences of significant health problems have lower utilization rates for screening services than healthier higher socioeconomic groups.[26] Papanicolaou screening has been demonstrated to be an effective technique for detecting early cervical carcinoma and adenosis.[31] Unfortunately, however, women over forty, who are at high risk, are less likely to be screened than younger women who are at lower risk.[32]

Finally, inadequate understanding of some test results compromises the effectiveness of screening. An example is the case of early screening for phenylketonuria (PKU) in infants. When such screening was mandated by law in many states, it was not realized that nine out of ten elevated PKU tests were transient and, thus, falsely positive.[33] Furthermore, it was not realized that the diet given PKU patients to protect them against brain damage from elevated phenylalanine could, itself, cause brain damage. More than 1000 cases of diet-induced brain damage have been reported.[34]

PATIENT EDUCATION AND SELF-CARE

Several studies have indicated that improved understanding of an illness by a patient and by the patient's family results in increased compliance with therapy and reduced numbers of complications.[35,36,37,38] These studies, although limited to specific groups of patients, strongly argue for the importance of patient education and of good communication between the patient and the physician. Surveys of practicing physicians, however, suggest that doctors feel that they do not have enough time to educate patients on all aspects of a disease or medications.[39,40] Moreover, they point to problems created by the patients' use of denial in dealing with their conditions.

There is little evidence that public education changes lifestyles or brings patients with specific symptoms to medical attention.[41] The low effectiveness of the national efforts to encourage smoking cessation and of the American Cancer Society's campaign to promulgate the seven signs of cancer are examples.[42]

It remains to be seen, however, whether widespread, intensive public or patient education can result in improved outcomes sufficient to justify the effort and costs involved.[40,43] Careful evaluation of such programs should be a prerequisite to their implementation.

Likewise, the values of self-diagnosis and self-treatment remain unclear. Countless millions of dollars are spent yearly on remedies for headaches, nervousness, and constipation, and on folk remedies and appliances. A number of books and manuals are available that encourage self-care, some written by physicians.[44] Still, the health benefits of these measures have never been well documented; and even if they should be shown to be beneficial, the risks of misinterpretation and of delayed diagnosis of potentially serious conditions may detract from or even negate any benefits.[8,45]

Self-care in the home under professional guidance is a different situation and has been used effectively for selected diseases; Parkinson's disease, diabetes mellitus, and hemophilia are a few examples.[40,45,46,47,48] In some areas, home care equipment is available at minimal cost on a shared basis to families of handicapped patients.[49]

HOME CARE

Blue Cross has been supporting the early discharge, home care programs on a limited basis.[50] In Rochester, New York, this program reported over $800,000 in savings by early discharge in 1972, and today, more than $2.5 million are being saved yearly.[51]

Most physicians, however, remain ignorant or skeptical about home care services.[52,53] In Toledo, Ohio, over 80 percent of the physicians were unaware that the early discharge, home care program was available to them in 1977. In most of the hospitals the nursing supervisors were also unaware of the existence of the program. The director of the community nursing service remarked that ignorance remains the major stumbling block to optimal implementation of home care programs.

Oddly enough, house calls by physicians can be cost effective in selected areas.[3] In some rural communities and in selected densely populated areas, house calls actually can be more economical than office visits. Patients must be carefully selected, however. In most modern practices, house calls would not be feasible. House calls by other professionals, such as visiting nurses, physician assistants, or other health associates, are available in many communities and are underutilized by most practicing physicians.

NONPHYSICIAN PRACTITIONERS

Nurse associates or practitioners and physician assistants have been proposed as less costly providers of primary care.[14,54] At the present time, however, while they are extenders of care, they also appear to be extenders of cost. Many studies have shown that they are well accepted by many physicians and by patients; perhaps they are better accepted by middle-class and upper-class patients than by the poor.[55] A study of the use of nurse practitioners in Burlington, Ontario, found that even though they worked well, they did not save money.[56] Under optimal circumstances physician assistants and nurse practitioners can be used to increase the volume of a practice and to save the physician from uncomplicated procedures, but few physicians are trained to work with such personnel effectively.

Nurse practitioners have also been used in rural areas where physicians either did not want to go or where it was uneconomical for them to go. Many problems and questions have arisen about the quality and supervision of the care provided under these circumstances. Clearly, these issues need to be more carefully evaluated.[24]

AMBULATORY SURGERY

It has been estimated that ambulatory surgery could save $6 to 15 billion a year in the United States with proper selection of surgical patients and with the ready availability of hospital support services.[57] The technology is available, support services are available, and many short-term surgery centers have been set up around the country.[50] In Kingston, Jamaica, over 5000 outpatient surgeries are performed each year on children with no mortality and no increased morbidity when compared to that experienced in hospitals in the same country.[58] For selected cases, such as herniorrhaphy, minor surgery on the skin, vasectomy, tonsillectomy, and placement of ear tubes, outpatient surgery can significantly reduce the cost of care by avoiding hospitalization.

CONCLUSION

The components of the ambulatory care system must be coordinated with each other and with the inpatient sector if maximal cost effectiveness of the health care system is to be realized. Moreover, the cost impact of each component must be assessed in relation to each other and to the system as a whole. Physicians in private practice still deliver the majority of ambulatory services; are they being trained to provide the services in an economical fashion? Are they being trained to understand or have experience with the resources available to them as alternatives to hospitalization? Can they utilize and trust other health professionals in the delivery of health care, whether they be nurse practitioners, nurse midwives, or physician assistants? Finally, can they feel secure in adapting to changes in practice procedures such as ambulatory surgery?

In the answers to these questions will lie much of the potential for cost containment in ambulatory care.

REFERENCES

1. Schweitzer, S. O. Cost effectiveness of early detection of disease. *Health Serv. Res.*, 22, 1974.
2. Reinhardt, U. E. Physician Productivity and the Demand for Health Manpower: An Economic Analysis. Cambridge, Mass., Ballinger, 1975.
3. Monsma, G. N. Marginal revenue and the demand for physicians' services. In H. E. Klarman (ed.), *Empirical Studies in Health Economics*. Baltimore, Johns Hopkins Press, 1970, p. 145.
4. Berarducci, A. A., et al. The teaching hospital and primary care. *N. Engl. J. Med.*, 292:615, 1975.
5. Gururaj, V. J., et al. Short stay in an outpatient department: An alternative to hospitalization. *Amer. J. Dis. Child.*, 123:128, 1972.
6. Hochheiser, L. I., et al. Effectiveness of the neighborhood health center on the use of pediatric emergency departments in Rochester, New York. *N. Engl. J. Med.*, 285:148, 1971.
7. Roemer, M. I., et al. Medical costs in relation to the organization of ambulatory health care. *N. Engl. J. Med.*, 280:988, 1969.
8. Donabedian, A. *Benefits in Medical Care Programs*. Cambridge, Mass., Harvard University Press, 1976.
9. Fuchs, V. R., and Kramer, M. J. *Determinants of Expenditures for Physicians' Services in the United States 1948-1968*. Washington, D.C., Government Printing Office, Publication No. (HSM) 73-3017, 1973.
10. *ALPHA: Planning for Ambulatory Care: Guideline for Future Development.* Syracuse, N.Y., Areawide and Local Planning for Health Action, Inc., 1974.
11. Bair, C. W. *Hospital Utilization in Toledo, Ohio, 1974-1977.* Report to HPA Northwest Ohio, 1977.
12. Wennberg, J., and Gittelsohn, A. Small area variations in health care delivery. *Science*, 182:1102, 1973.
13. Walsh, R. J., Aherne, P., Ryan, G. A. (eds.:). *The Profile of Medical Practice*. Chicago, A.M.A., 1972.
14. Pless, I. B.: The changing face of primary pediatrics. *Pediatr. Clin. N. Amer.*, 21:223, 1974.
15. Bergman, A. B., et al. Time and motion study of practicing pediatricians. *Pediatrics*, 38:254, 1966.
16. Drachman, R. H., et al. Computers and ambulatory health services. *Adv. Pediatr.*, 20:101, 1973.
17. Sims, N. H., et al. Self evaluation in ambulatory care. *Adv. Pediatr.*, 20:177, 1973.

18. Elwood, P. M. Alternatives to regulation: Improving the market. In *Controls on Health Care.* Washington, National Academy of Sciences, 1975, p. 49.
19. Elnick, R. A. Substitution of outpatient for inpatient hospital care: A cost analysis. *Inquiry*, 13:245, 1976.
20. Ginzberg, E. Paradoxes and trends: An economist looks at health care. *N. Engl. J. Med.*, 296:814, 1977.
21. Roghmann, K. J., et al. Anticipated and actual effects of medicaid on the medical-care pattern of children. *N. Engl. J. Med.*, 285:1053, 1971.
22. Fuchs, V. R.: *Who Shall Live: Health Economics and Social Choice.* New York, Basic Books, 1974.
23. Hurwitz, R. A., et al. Impact of intensive training on diagnosis of cardiac murmurs. Abstracts, Ambulatory Pediatric Association, 16th Annual Meeting, 1976, p. 17.
24. Yankauer, A. Standards of health care. *Amer. J. Pub. Health*, 59:1104, 1969.
25. Whitby, L. G. Screening for disease; definitions and criteria. *Lancet*, 2:819–821, 1974.
26. Collen, M. F. Periodic health examinations. *Primary Care*, 2:197, 1976.
27. Dales, L. G., et al. Evaluation of periodic multiphasic health checkup. *Meth. Inform. Med.*, 13:140, 1970.
28. A.M.A. News, May 11, 1977, p. 8.
29. Sane, S. M., et al. Value of preoperative chest x-ray examinations in children. *Pediatrics*, 60:699, 1977.
30. Collen, M. F. Dollar cost per positive test for automated multiphasic screening. *N. Engl. J. Med.*, 283:459, 1970.
31. Martin, P. L. How preventable is invasive cervical cancer? A community study of preventive factors. *Amer. J. Obstet. Gynecol.*, 113:541, 1972.
32. Dickinson, L., et al. Evaluation of the effectiveness of cytological screening for cervical cancer. II. Survival parameters before and after inception of screening. *Mayo Clin. Proc.*, 47:545, 1972.
33. American Academy of Pediatrics, Committee on the Handicapped Child. Phenylketonuria and the phenylalanienemias of infancy. *Pediatrics*, 49:628, 1972.
34. Cost-benefit analysis of newborn screening for metabolic disorders. *N. Engl. J. Med.*, 291:1414, 1974.
35. Green, L. W., et al. Clinical trials of health education for hypertensive patients: Design and baseline data. *Prev. Med.*, 4:417, 1975.
36. Gordis, L. Effectiveness of comprehensive-care programs in preventing rheumatic fever. *N. Engl. J. Med.*, 289:331, 1973.
37. Rosenberg, S. Patient education leads to better care for heart patients. *HSMHA Health Rep.*, 86:793, 1971.
38. Somers, A. R. Task Force Report. Health promotion and consumer health education. In *Preventive Medicine, U.S.A.* New York, Prodist, 1976.
39. Francis, V., et al. Gaps in doctor-patient communication. *N. Engl. J. Med.*, 280:535, 1969.
40. Green, L. Toward cost-benefit evaluations of health education: Some concepts, methods, and examples. *Health Education Monographs*, Vol. 2 suppl., p. 34, 1974.

41. Wade, S. Trends in public knowledge about health and illness. *Am. J. Pub. Health*, 60:485, 1970.
42. Haggerty, R. J. Changing lifestyles to improve health. *Prev. Med.*, 6:276, 1977.
43. Rocella, E. J. Potential for reducing health care costs by public and patient education. *Pub. Health Rep.*, 91:223, 1976.
44. Vickery, D. M., and Fries, J. F. *Take Care of Yourself.* Reading, Mass., Addison-Wesley, 1976.
45. Green, L., et al. Research and demonstration issues in self-care: Measuring the decline of medicocentrism. Conference on Self-Care Programs, Rockville, Maryland, National Center for Health Services Research, 1976, p. 14.
46. Katz, H., and Clauch, R. Accuracy of a home throat culture program: A study of parent participation in health care. *Pediatrics*, 53:961, 1974.
47. Pednault, E. Home care of patients with Parkinson's disease. *Primary Care*, 4:485, 1977.
48. Bell, J. Self-care aids for the Parkinsonian patient and his family. *Primary Care*, 4:449, 1977.
49. Green, M. Innovative methods of expanding ambulatory services. *Adv. Pediatr.*, 20:15, 1973.
50. Cloud, D. T., et al. The surgicenter: A fresh concept in outpatient surgery. *K. Pediatr. Surg.*, 7:206, 1972.
51. Boulay, R., and White, D. W. New home-care thrust: The Rochester model. *Patient Care*, Jan. 1974, p. 133.
52. Bergman, A. B., et al. A pediatric home care program in London: Ten year experience. *Pediatrics*, 36:314, 1965.
53. Bluestone, N. Organized home care—now that it's been "discovered," who'll make it work? *Mod. Med.*, Mar. 1977, p. 41.
54. Clow, C. L., et al. Management of hereditary metabolic diseases: Role of allied health personnel. *N. Engl. J. Med.*, 283:459, 1970.
55. Conant, J., et al. Anticipated patient acceptance of new nursing roles and physicians' assistants. *Am. J. Dis. Child.*, 122:202, 1971.
56. Spitzer, W. O., et al. The Burlington randomized trial of the nurse practitioner. *N. Engl. J. Med.*, 290:251–256, 1974.
57. Kernaghan, S. G. Peripheral issues cloud basic questions in day surgery. *Hospitals*, 49:58, 1975.
58. El-Shafie, M., and Shapiro, R. P. Outpatient pediatric surgery in a developing country. *Pediatrics*, 60:600, 1977.

Chapter 4

Efficient Office Practice

William Y. Rial*

High-quality medical care, like anything else of high quality, is high-cost care. Beyond a certain point, a rationing of funds inevitably results in a rationing of the quality of, or access to, medical care. The real issue, then, is how to reach that point without going beyond it. In this book much needed attention is not only focused on realistic, rather than cosmetic, approaches to cost containment of medical care, but also it is recognized that the private sector should carry the primary responsibility for implementing these approaches. Many practical and effective methods of promoting more *efficient office practice* have been gathered and widely disseminated by the AMA through its Department of Practice Management. In this chapter these methods are discussed.

We estimate that by increasing efficiency, office practice costs can be reduced by as much as 5 percent. Because solo practices, partnerships, and small groups are still the predominant forms of medical practice in this country, even a savings of 5 percent may represent a respectable total. This is precisely why the AMA, during 1977, conducted 161 practice management workshops for physicians and office assistants across the nation. These workshops serve to

*Speaker, House of Delegates, American Medical Association.

underscore a variety of methods of increasing the efficiency of office practice.

Medical Office Records

One area of office practice often found to be in need of greater efficiency is medical record keeping. The efficient filing and retrieval of medical records obviously can considerably reduce time and labor costs. A number of practical methods are available to achieve this goal. *Date stamping* is one solution. It consists of indicating numerically, on the outside of each patient's file folder, the year the folder was first compiled and the dates of activities in succeeding years. Inactive files can thereby be weeded out, and the active files kept lean. Date stamping is easy to do, costs almost nothing, and can be used with any type of medical record system.

Next is *color coding*. The basic purpose of color coding is to prevent misfiling of patient charts, although it also can speed up filing and retrieval. A number of color coding systems, some quite sophisticated, have been developed in large group practices and in hospitals where thousands of records must be stored. However, there is a growing trend toward the use of color coding even in small practices, with the selection of a particular system based on singular wants and needs. Physicians have found that proper *file equipment* can increase efficiency. Shelf files or circular files, for example, can provide space saving benefits as well as operating efficiencies over the old cabinet or multidrawer files.

File folders can also add to efficiency. Today, the use of larger, 9-½- by 12-inch file folders has become almost standardized. The larger folder helps reduce what often is called the "fat file" or overstuffed files characteristic of smaller folders. The larger folders, together with a more efficient organization of the material in the patient record, result in significant savings of the physician's time when seeking specific information about a patient to facilitate followup of chronic problems. Although the switch to larger folders can be a tedious task, it will more than repay the effort in the long run. A *disease cross-index* file may be used only a few times a year, but when needed, it literally can save hours of search time. The cost is minimal, and when a new patient chart is being compiled or when a new diagnosis is established, it takes less than 60 seconds to make the appropriate entry on the disease cross-index card.

Viewed strictly from an efficiency standpoint, the physician who makes the *actual record entry* immediately after patient examination from a standup desk generally will gain a few minutes over the physician who does charts sitting down. The physician who dictates the patient records is probably the most efficient of all. In fact, an increasing number of physicians are dictating medical records because of the development of relatively inexpensive dictating equipment and because of the greater legibility of resulting records. The time savings from dictating, of course, need to be balanced against the additional expense of transcribing.

Finally, *patient history questionnaires* not only are time savers for the physician but also may help improve the quality of care. They can be particularly effective at the time of an initial examination or subsequent complete reexaminations to provide an up-to-date data base for each patient. The questionnaire results should be located in a clearly identifiable part of the medical record where they will be readily accessible for reference.

Patient Education

Patient information booklets are strongly recommended by practice management consultants. Developed by and for a particular office practice, they provide information such as office hours, type of practice, number of physicians in the group, services available, fees, and payment procedures. Although the primary purpose of these booklets is better patient relations, it has been found that they reduce nonproductive phone calls by as much as 30 percent.

Disease-oriented patient education materials can be used to help patients better understand their particular medical problem and thereby assist the physician in its treatment. This type of material, which may consist of pamphlets, fact sheets, or audio-visual devices, for example, can save the physician a great deal of repetitious, time-consuming explanation to patients. To be maximally effective, however, such materials should both be practical and constructive in their contents and take into account language, education, and cultural characteristics of patients.

Appointment Schedules

The so-called *modified-wave appointment system* seems to help the physician make more efficient use of time than the standard appointment book marked off in fifteen-minute segments. Under the modified-wave system, a physician may simultaneously schedule three or four patients at the beginning of each hour. While the physician examines the first patient, office assistants are preparing the other patients for examination in adjacent examining rooms. The final ten or fifteen minutes of each hour are left open. This system offers three major advantages over the fifteen-minute interval method. First, if a patient fails to show up, or is late, the physician has other patients to treat. Second, the use of office assistants to perform the more routine examination procedures increases efficiency and tends to reduce overall patient waiting time. Third, the likelihood of long waits by patients is reduced; and finally, the modified-wave system permits the appointment schedule to be tailor-made to a particular office practice. Schedules thus can reflect variations in the specialties of the physicians involved, personal working habits, the number and skills of allied health personnel, and the physical facilities involved such as the number of examining rooms and diagnostic equipment. Design of the system requires physicians and their office assistants to devote considerable thought to the special needs of their practices. This works not only to the benefit of the provider, but to the benefit of the patient as well. The developer of this system is Dr. Walter Lane, a physician whose background includes industrial engineering. Fundamentally, he used time and motion data to develop the model appointment system, which he then called the modified-wave system.

Patient scheduling, of course, consists of much more than entering names in an appointment book. Flexibility to account for emergencies, the need to recall some patients, and patient mix all need to be considered. A physician with a larger percentage of elderly patients may have to set aside more time for each patient, while routine postoperative examinations may require less time. Every office practice should have a patient flow system that makes allowances for such variations.

Efficient Use of a Physician's Time

Anything that helps the physician improve productivity and efficiency helps reduce the costs of care provided to each patient. Unfortunately, however, the efficient use of a physician's time is extremely difficult to measure accurately. Business executives, for example, can keep a time log for a few days or weeks, compare the results in relation to defined goals, and readjust their schedules accordingly. They may decide to deal with difficult sales and production problems in the morning when they are fresh and complete routine tasks in the afternoon. Practicing physicians, however, are slaves as well as masters of their patient appointment schedules, because patients, and the infinitely variable medical problems that afflict them, are not easily fitted into precise time slots. Demands for physician time and skills cannot always be reliably predicted in advance. Furthermore, subjective values such as patient dignity and satisfaction must be taken into account, especially since there can be no guaranteed results. A physician, therefore, can be highly successful and "process" sixty patients a day, only to be considered a failure because of patients who are disgruntled or inadequately served as a result of assembly-line techniques. What the average physician can do, however, is to minimize wasted time and effort by developing a patient appointment system that is both realistic and flexible and then attempting to adhere to it as much as possible.

Efficient Use of Office Assistants

Allied health personnel and administrative personnel should be employed in such a way as to maximize use of their capabilities. Clearly, the delegation of nonmedical tasks to administrative assistants is cost efficient. The participation of administrative assistants in practice-management workshops such as those sponsored by the AMA can only add to this efficiency. But the *delegation of medical tasks* is another matter entirely, since patient health, safety, and satisfaction are directly at stake. Medical procedures that currently are being delegated range from the routine, such as the dressing of minor wounds and the taking of blood pressures, to more complicated procedures, such as the taking of patient histories, the performing of routine physical examinations and pelvic examinations, and the followup of patients with stable chronic diseases such as hypertension and diabetes mellitus. The extent to which any, or all, such tasks are delegated depends on a variety of factors; for example, the exercise of the physician's judgment and confidence in such delegation; the skills, training, and experience of the allied health personnel involved; and their willingness to assume added responsibilities. The policy ultimately adopted, therefore, should conform to the singular capabilities found in a particular office practice.

The importance of patient satisfaction cannot be overemphasized. For example, if an allied health professional performs a medical procedure, especially a nonroutine procedure, and a complication ensues, the patient may be more likely to feel that the physician has been negligent and to file a malpractice suit. In fact, patient satisfaction, must be considered in all of the approaches to more efficient office practice outlined in this chapter. On the one hand, patient satisfaction is important because a positive attitude on the part of the patient may be at least as important a medical outcome as a good technical result; on the other hand, it is important because of the very real risk that *dissatisfaction* may lead to complex and costly liability insurance problems. As Dr. Edmund D. Pellegrino, the noted American physician and teacher, has said, "[The physician] must guard against the dehumanization so easily and inadvertently perpetrated by a group in the name of efficiency." Certainly, patients today are telling physicians that they want caring for, as well as curing, with more emphasis on the caring. The truly efficient physician takes time to treat patients in spirit as well as body and ensures that the office assistants do likewise. It is *this* kind of efficiency, in fact, that leads to treatment of the whole patient and to medical care of truly high quality.

AMBULATORY CARE AND COST CONTROL

Some physicians believe that it is inappropriate to focus the entire responsibility for cost control on physicians. Government, third-party payers, hospitals, and patients all affect medical care costs and must share the responsibility. Thus, the relationship of practice variations to cost control as well as strategies for facilitating cost control must be considered.

Practice Variations and Cost Control

Before corrective actions can be taken, it is felt that it is necessary to determine why there are variations in the cost of care provided by different physicians. Indiscriminate efforts to reduce medical care costs, without first achieving an adequate understanding of the factors influencing those costs, might incur the risks of decreased quality of care and of antagonism from the profession.

Reasons for Practice Variations

1. Physicians may practice differently because of the lack of documentation that one practice pattern is superior to another. For example, some physicians are more likely than others to refer patients with angina pectoris for coronary artery bypass graft surgery. At present, data are insufficient to define clearly appropriate indications for surgery.

2. In other cases, sufficient data may be available but the practicing physician may be unaware of it.
3. It is also likely that, even though physicians have access to the same data, they may arrive at different decisions because of differences in problem-solving techniques used.
4. Personal attributes of the physician such as age, specialty, board certification, and training influence the use of clinical resources.
5. Behavior of physicians often may be governed by recent experiences, even though these experiences are not necessarily representative. Outcomes of recent cases, therefore, may strongly influence the management of current cases.
6. Personal monetary gain probably does influence physician behavior, but considerable disagreement exists over the degree to which this is so. Achieving a target income may also be an important goal for many physicians.
7. Self-referral for laboratory testing and radiologic examinations are cited as areas that are particularly susceptible to abuse. Data indicate that utilization rates for these services may be double in situations where the possibility of self-referral exists.
8. Unnecessary repeat examinations are ordered during hospitalizations either because ambulatory records are unavailable or because hospitals refuse to accept the results of tests performed outside. Physicians and hospitals are felt to share responsibility for this problem and for its solution.
9. The setting in which physicians practice is felt to strongly influence the way they practice. Most striking are differences between utilization rates in prepaid and fee-for-service practices. Some, however, question whether physicians practicing in prepaid practices might be different types of physicians from those in fee-for-service practices. Differences, such as urban versus rural and community hospital versus teaching hospital, are also felt to influence practice style and resultant costs.
10. A physician's own workload may influence behavior. Busy physicians, for example, are felt to order more tests in order to expedite evaluation of their patients.
11. Fear of malpractice suits may influence a physician's behavior and induce the practice of defensive medicine and, hence, excessive use of diagnostic tests. It is noteworthy, however, that only 2 to 3 percent of malpractice cases are related to the nonperformance of laboratory examinations.

Assessment of Practice Variations

It is felt that information currently available is insufficient to document the importance of the possible reasons for practice variations and the degree to which each contributes to medical care costs. In fact, it is possible that these variations may represent a healthy, pluralistic mix of alternative styles of practice rather than a significant problem. Profile analyses of different practices, carefully controlled for possible confounding variables, need to be performed in both intra- and interinstitutional formats. Practices with wide variations in utilization rates should then become the subjects of medical staff discussions, and individual practice outlyers should be approached to determine the reasons for their outlyer status. Investigations should focus on the use of ancillary services, both diagnostic and therapeutic, and on office visit and hospitalization rates.

Case mix is acknowledged as a critical variable that needs to be taken into account. When the causes for variations have been defined and their contributions to unnecessary medical care costs evaluated, strategies for cost control can be devised in a cause-specific manner. For some causes, such as physician ignorance of cost-effective decision-making techniques, education may be an appropriate solution; for others, such as differences in practice settings, institutional changes may be required; and for still others, financial incentives and disincentives for the physician may have to be developed.

Strategies for Cost Control

1. *System monitoring of health care services,* in the form of utilization review and external and internal audits, or both, not only can help to bring to light instances of fraud and abuse, but also can be used as an educational tool to encourage cost-effective decision making. The results of an EMCRO (Experimental Medical Care Review Organization) project at Johns Hopkins suggested that outcome audits, but not process audits, were correlated with the quality of care. If quality of care is the objective, therefore, emphasis should be put on outcome audits. The determination of audit criteria should not be the province of a single specialty but should be the responsibility of all involved specialties. For example, if an audit is to deal with the use of a particular type of x ray, both internists and radiologists should have inputs.

Similarly, the expertise of clinical pathologists should be sought when criteria are being established for the appropriate use of particular laboratory tests. National guidelines for appropriate utilization should be established, and they could then serve as points of reference for narrowing variations in practice.

2. *Coordination of services* provided to individual patients should be emphasized. Better coordination of care for the ambulatory patient who requires the input from multiple specialties as well as the coordination of ambulatory care and inpatient care are involved. The concept of the primary physician as the coordinator of all referrals and elective hospitalizations may have considerable merit. In this role the primary physician can provide a significant deterrent effect on excessive use of health resources, particularly if he or she has a financial incentive to do so, such as in prepaid practices or other arrangements in which cost sharing is involved. The availability of ambulatory office records and laboratory examinations to the hospital and acceptance of these studies by the hospital would also help to avoid the considerable reduplication of services that now accompanies hospitalization. Close communication between the hospital physician and ambulatory physician (if they are different) is another prerequisite to effective coordination of services.

3. The use of *efficient management techniques* and judicious use of management consultants could achieve considerable savings. Appropriate delegation of responsibility, patient scheduling, medical records, and financial accounting are some areas that require attention.

4. The importance of encouraging physicians to be *aware of the costs* of medical care is repeatedly emphasized as being of utmost importance. Education in costs and cost-effective decision making should begin in medical school. Continuing medical education, peer pressure, and inclusion of cost considerations in licensure and relicensure examinations and in medical care audits are suggested as ways to increase cost awareness.

5. *Substitution of ambulatory care for hospital care* in situations where this is appropriate should be an important objective. The availability of ambulatory facilities for diagnostic studies and for surgery is one component; the restructuring of health insurance coverage packages to reduce incentives to hospitalize patients and to include fuller coverage of ambulatory ser-

vices and adjustment of reimbursement levels for different medical services is another. Current reimbursement levels favor surgical and diagnostic procedures over services that require medical judgment and communication with patients. An argument can be made that prices should be based on the skills, time, and effort of the practitioner rather than on historical precedent, as is the case at present. Financial incentives created by adjustment of reimbursement levels will encourage young physicians to choose primary care specialties over other specialties that are currently represented in excess; they will also discourage excessive use of diagnostic and surgical technologies and will encourage the physician to spend more time with the individual patient than now is possible. More time, in turn, will allow greater emphasis on the caring functions of medicine, better patient education, and better preventive health services.

6. *Financial incentives* for the cost-effective use of medical services may take several forms. Emphasis on cost-sharing types of medical practice organization such as prepaid medical practices is one. Another incentive, which would also apply to fee-for-service practices, might include providing a financial reward to physicians who decrease their use of ancillary services. Such a plan is being tested in a pilot program by Michigan Blue Shield.

7. *A coinsurance provision* should be included in any national health insurance program. The consensus was that this would have a significant influence in curtailing use of health services that provide small marginal benefits to patients. If the coinsurance mechanism were progressive, it would not be likely to reduce significantly the access of the poor to health care.

8. Regulations to *limit self-referral* for laboratory and radiologic procedures would have a favorable effect not only on costs, but also on the quality of care because of the difficulties of maintaining quality control in many small privately run laboratories.

9. *Second-opinion programs* for elective surgical procedures were felt to have limited potential for cost savings. In many instances it would be preferable to obtain the second opinion from a physician with a specialty different from that of the first physician. For example, a cardiologist for cardiac surgery; or a neurosurgeon for a low-back syndrome for whom an orthopedist recommends surgery.

10. The global fee was felt to have considerable potential for controlling costs. This kind of fee has been in existence for obstetrical services for many years. Its expansion to include other medical and surgical services should be considered. Some of its major advantages would be to limit the lengths of hospitalizations and the unnecessary use of ancillary services.

PART III

Inpatient Care

Chapter 5

Variations in Inpatient Care

*Duncan Neuhauser**

We will review variation in hospital practice and its implications for the costs of inpatient care, thereby suggesting, we hope, avenues for thought and inquiry.

That possibilities for cost savings exist should not be a criticism of the medical profession today. In the last twenty years, medicine has been responding to the public's desire for more medical research and the desire that the new and often expensive care be available to all without regard for the patient's ability to pay. Medicine has responded. Now we are discovering that this expanded care is costly, and a new concern about costs is being raised. Very likely medicine will respond to this concern. When viewed in this way, it should be no criticism of medicine today that costs of medical care are high. If medicine does not respond in the next decade, criticism may then be appropriate.

Conceptually, inpatient care can be divided into several components. Preadmission, admission, length of stay, diagnostic and treatment inputs, and discharge and postdischarge. These stages are stated in Table 5.1 and form the outline and structure of the following review of their cost implications.

*Associate Professor of Health Services Administration, Harvard School of Public Health. From September 1979, Professor of Community Health, School of Medicine, Case Western Reserve University.

Table 5.1. The Cost-related Components of Inpatient Care

---

1. Preadmission care (testing)
2. The decision to admit
3. Average length of stay
4. Diagnostic inputs
5. Treatment inputs
6. Criteria for patient discharge
7. Posthospital and long-term care

PREADMISSION CARE (TESTING)

By testing before admission rather than after admission, presumably the patient's stay will be shortened and money saved. One recent study suggested that modest savings were possible.[1] Their importance, however, was limited by the following factors:

1. Preadmission testing is limited in usefulness, primarily to elective admissions.
2. It does not always reduce patient stay. It may simply mean that the patient is admitted at six in the evening rather than ten in the morning. If a patient day is billed on the basis of the midnight census, this technique will not affect length of stay or the patient's room rate bill.
3. Third-party payers have been careful about entering this area in order to make their financial payout predictable. They do not wish to cover *all* outpatient testing in order to gain the comparatively small savings that result from preadmission testing.

THE DECISION TO ADMIT

Of all cost-saving approaches to medical care, the decision not to admit a patient to a hospital creates the greatest potential savings. We come to this conclusion by observing the great variation in admission rates per 1000 population from one place to another and from one type of provider to another.

Fixed versus Variable Costs

Of all hospital costs a high percentage are fixed costs and a low percentage variable costs. Fixed costs, in the jargon of accounting and economics, are costs that occur whether or not a service or product is produced. For the hospital, the building, heat, electricity, equipment, and the salaries of personnel have to be paid whether the occupancy rate is 40 percent, 60 percent, 80 percent, or 100 percent. These are fixed costs. The higher the occupancy rate, the more the revenue for the voluntary U.S. hospital. If most of the costs are fixed, the hospital has every reason to maintain high occupancy. Variable costs are costs that are used for each patient day. An additional patient means a few more x-ray films, three more meals consumed, slightly more laboratory reagents, greater wear on the sheets, and a few more disposable syringes used.

This basic phenomenon is the fundamental driving force that influences voluntary hospitals. Keep the beds filled! The more beds filled, the more likely it is that revenue will exceed expenses. The surplus can then be plowed back into expanding services and building more beds in hopes that this will attract more doctors to the staff and still more patients to keep the occupancy rate up. Thus the cycle continues. The certificate of need and hospital planning laws attempt to slow this snowballing effect.

The physician is often pressured by the administration to keep the beds filled. When the hospital beds are filled and the waiting list long, utilization review can be pursued with great enthusiasm. However, when summer comes and occupancy falls this enthusiasm may diminish.

International Comparisons

Variations in hospital admission rates between different countries are considerable. Admission rates per 1000 population per year for eight countries are shown in Table 5.2. The Soviet Union has more and England fewer admissions than we do.[2,3] It seems hard to ex-

Table 5.2. Admissions to General Hospitals per 1000 Population per Year for Selected Countries (1969)[3]

Soviet Union	169
Sweden	147
United States	145
West Germany	112
England and Wales	100
Italy	98.5
Netherlands	92
France	71

plain these large differences other than by historical circumstances and medical custom,[4] and Table 5.2 does not even show the extremes. Saskatchewan, Canada, has 214 admissions compared to our 145.[5] Are U.S. patients made to suffer because fewer are admitted to the hospital than in Saskatchewan? Probably not. Even though England has a lower admission rate, observers report that about 35 percent of patients in British hospitals do not need to be there.[3]

This finding suggests that 65 admissions per 1000 population per year would be appropriate, a rate that is 45 percent of the American admission rate.

British planners long ago discovered that a hospital bed, if available, is used, and that admissions can be reduced and costs controlled only by limiting the number of beds. Tight control of beds has been one of the cornerstones of British medical planning.[6] Increasingly, in the United States one hears health planners call for a reduction in the number of hospital beds. However, closing hospital beds has been a near political impossibility in the United States. Attempts to close the smallest obstetrical units, let alone entire community hospitals, meet with vigorous community opposition. One of the few countries that has been able to reduce the number of hospital beds significantly is the Republic of Ireland. It reduced its number of beds by 40 percent from 1959 to 1968.[3] Are the lower admission rates associated with reduced numbers of hospital beds good or bad? The answer is a resounding "maybe."

In a sense each country gets the medical service it deserves. A country's medical care system evolves out of a political, historical, legal, economic, and cultural context. What is a fine idea for England may be inappropriate for the United States and vice versa. English patients are often content to wait for a year or two to get varicose veins surgically treated while American patients would be outraged by such delays. The English public is appalled that Americans must pay for their medical care directly, whereas Americans accept this. The list of differences between countries could go on and on.

All too often a comparison of medical care between the United States and elsewhere is used for political polemics. Political critics of American medicine are likely to start their Jeremiad by saying that people in some other countries live longer than we do. Political critics of national health insurance in the United States will use any aspect of the British National Health Service that they do not like to condemn an expanded role for the U.S. government in medicine. Such approaches are objectionable to dedicated medical professionals everywhere. Dispassionate inquiry, possibly along the following lines, will achieve greater rewards:

1. The use of international comparisons to reinforce the realization that medical care can be delivered in very different ways.[7]
2. There is usually a reason for these differences. A fruitful approach is to ask why these differences occur.
3. A given country's medical care system is not necessarily all of one piece. One might decide, for example, that home care in Great Britain is excellent but that British hospitals are too often old and antiquated. We need to look at the trees as well as the forests.
4. Approach international comparisons with the idea that whatever we decide to do in America will fit our unique genius and reflect our own follies too. This means that it is very difficult to import another country's way of doing things wholesale. It probably will not fit here.

Health Maintenance Organizations and Hospital Admissions

Much has been written on this topic. For an early review see Greenlick[8,9] and for a more recent detailed study see Gaus.[10] The Gaus study examined ten HMOs and two foundations and found significant differences from controls only in the rates of hospital utilization (Table 5.3). No differences were noted in the previous health status of patients, and no differences were found in either the use of ambulatory care or "preventive" care.

A similar pattern of hospital utilization is reported by Dr. Shalowitz for enrollees in his health plan from two large Chicago employers in Chapter 6.

Table 5.3. Use of General Hospitals in Different Medical Care Systems[10]

	Admissions per 1000 Persons	Average Length of Stay	Days of Care per 1000 Population
HMOs	46	7.4	340
Controls	114	7.7	880
Foundations	106	5.8	610
Controls	122	4.5	548

The Double Standard: How Society Exploits the Altruism of Physicians

What follows is half in jest and half entirely serious.

Consider the longshoreman. Once upon a time the unloading of ships was a long, slow process. Boxes, barrels, and bales, piled in the hold of a freighter, were picked up and stacked by hand on platforms that were hoisted out of the ship onto the dock where forklift trucks would move them into sheds for future loading onto trucks or boxcars. Then came container cargo ships. Cargo was placed in large sealed containers shaped like the boxes on big highway trucks. They could be unloaded faster with a fraction of the crew of longshoremen. This change greatly increased productivity and reduced costs. Before unions would agree to this change, however, they insisted that a large share of the savings should be passed on to longshoremen in the form of a 40 percent wage increase for those who would still be employed. This was agreed to and the changes made at a time when inflation was a major concern and other unions who were seeking mere 10 percent pay raises received "jawboning" by the president. The longshoremen's 40 percent pay raise was justified by the increased productivity.

Now think how this would apply to reduced hospital admissions if physicians thought like the longshoremen's union. Physicians would agree to reduce hospital admissions from 145 per 1000 to 95 per 1000 only if half the "savings" were returned to the physicians. If one assumes $50 billion spent on hospitals, this 34 percent reduction would be a savings of $17 billion, half of which would be $8.5 billion. If divided among 225,000 physicians, the yearly net incomes of each physician would increase about $40,000. We have yet to hear any physician talk in these terms. The regulators who aspire to reduce hospital utilization do not look at it this way. From the perspective of the longshoremen's union, the regulators are exploiting the altruism of physicians.

AVERAGE LENGTH OF STAY (ALOS)

Variations in the average length of stay in the hospital from one location to another have long been noted.[11,12,13,14,15,16] Patients stay in hospitals longer in New England than in California. This was true in 1976, and it was also true in 1950.[17,18] Why? In fact, California may have the world's shortest length of stay. The farther one gets from California the longer the average length of stay seems to be, and by the time one reaches Germany (18.5 days) and the Soviet Union (perhaps 17 to 19 days), it has doubled (see Table 5.4).

Differences in the length of stay by country for general hospitals[19] may be due to the same kinds of patients staying longer, a different mix of patients, different discharge criteria, or what is most likely, a combination of these factors. Swedish hospitals have similar lengths of stay for matched patients to the United States but contain more patients who would be in nursing homes in our country. It is reported that one reason for the long Soviet stay is that patients are discharged when they are ready to return to work. This is analogous to American military hospitals' discharge criterion of "fit for duty," which probably explains their longer length of stay.

Average Length of Stay and Costs

The shorter the average length of stay (ALOS), the lower the costs. This seemingly obvious relationship is not all that simple.

1. If other factors are held constant, as ALOS becomes shorter for a hospital, the costs per patient day go up because the same number of tests and treatments are squeezed into a shorter period of time.
2. As ALOS becomes shorter, the cost per case or per admission falls. This is true at least up to a point; too short a stay may lead to chaos as everything will be attempted in too short a time.[20]
3. These statements refer to similar patients in similar hospitals. One day in an intensive care unit in a large city hospital that costs $800 per day may cost as much as ten days in a twenty-bed rural hospital.

Table 5.4. Average Length of Stay (ALOS) in General Hospitals in Seven Countries (1969)[3]

	ALOS
United States	9.3 days
England and Wales	11.1
Sweden	12.6
Italy	13.4
Netherlands	17.9
France	18
West Germany	18.5

4. Shortening the length of stay may result in higher costs for third-party payers. If early discharge of recuperating surgical patients means that the beds will be filled by cardiac bypass surgery patients, the effect will be more patients cared for, higher per diem costs, and more total dollars paid by (say) Blue Cross. However, if shorter lengths of stay lead to a reduction in the number of hospital beds, the third-party payer will then pay out less money. If all this sounds like a tangle, it is, and it is only part of the cluster of problems surrounding medical care costs.

DIAGNOSTIC INPUTS

Physical examinations and medical histories, laboratory and x-ray tests, EKGs, and a variety of other testing techniques are included here. Whether to test or not is one of the questions that cost-effective clinical decision making can address effectively. Variations in the number of types of diagnostic tests for similar patients have been frequently observed.[21,22] Several examples have been discussed in earlier chapters.

The careful scheduling of diagnostic tests will help to speed up the diagnostic process, thence, to shorten the length of stay. For example, long hospital stays are frequently related to a backlog of work in radiology. Better scheduling, careful utilization review, and increased x-ray capacity are approaches to coping with this problem.

Another fruitful area of inquiry is repeated tests, urinalyses, cultures of various types, and electrolyte determinations, for example. Are repeated tests providing useful information? In one hospital the attending physicians had a great mistrust of the accuracy of the hospital's laboratory, and thus they were in the habit of ordering many tests twice to increase the "reliability" of results.

TREATMENT INPUTS

Quite a few diseases allow for alternative treatments that have clear cost implications. Medical treatment or cardiac bypass surgery for angina and dialysis or transplantation for kidney disease are two examples.

For some patients the choice is clear, but for others the choice is "close" and could go either way. If angina is severe enough or the left main coronary artery is involved, bypass surgery then appears to be the treatment of choice. But if angina is mild and medically controllable and the arterial occlusions are minimal, the choice might go either way. This choice for one patient could make a difference of about $15,000 of hospital expenditure. One study comparing HMO and non-HMO patients showed that the HMO patients (adjusted for age) had one-third the rate of cardiac bypass surgery as non-HMO patients.

This is not to say that one surgical rate is "better," than the other. However, we can conclude that the cost implications are considerable and that the variations are well worth examining. All of the following questions could be asked:

1. Are the HMO patients getting too little bypass surgery and missing out on its benefits?
2. Are the non-HMO patients getting too much bypass surgery?
3. How would you explain this difference to the third-party payers, the government, labor unions, and employers who are paying for it?
4. If these HMO patients get less care, perhaps they also pay less. An economist might say if people have a choice of paying more and getting more or paying less and getting less, there is nothing wrong with that. Do you agree?

Because American medical care is paid for in many ways and there is no agreement as to how it will be paid for in the future, we cannot even ask the "right" questions. There is no one right question to ask about medical care costs.

Controversy about alternative treatment forms is usually argued on the basis of medical benefits.[23] Many of these legitimate debates, however, could also be viewed as to their cost implications. Fetal monitoring, for example, a relatively inexpensive technique to monitor fetal distress during delivery, seems to have a side effect of increasing Caesarian section rates by perhaps 10 percent. The total effect, therefore, is to reduce the risk to the infant and increase the risk slightly for the mother, with increased cost all around. Another example is that of more or less extensive surgery for breast cancer (radical mastectomy versus modified radical mastectomy versus lumpectomy).[24] This legitimate debate has a number of interesting cost implications. Mammography screening, inpatient versus outpatient tissue biopsy, type of surgery, chemotherapy, and radiation therapy all have cost implications.

DISCHARGE CRITERIA

When is a patient ready to go home? Opinions vary, home circumstances vary, and patients vary. These variations have cost implications.

One of the better-known questions surrounds hospital discharge for acute myocardial infarction. Twenty-one days was once a standard, then it became two weeks, and now perhaps one week may be appropriate in selected patients. (McNeer et al. estimate that a seven-day stay could save from $360 to $435 million per year at 1977 prices for the country as a whole.)[25]

While on this issue of hospitalization for acute myocardial infarction, the fascinating puzzle of Mathur and coworkers should be addressed.[26] This randomized trial from Bristol, England, assigned patients to home care hospitalization. It was initially reported in 1971 and again in 1976,[26] the latter based on an expanded series. Mathur found no difference in survival for patients in the first study between the kinds of care given. It should be read first to look for possible questionable aspects of the study. The second report attempts to address many of these questions. In this expanded series there was no difference in survival for patients under age sixty. For patients aged sixty to seventy the home care patients lived longer, but the difference was statistically significant at the 10-percent level ($p < 10$). This difference could have occurred by chance less than one in ten times. If one accepts these findings, the implications for medical care costs is vast indeed.

This study appears to have had no impact in the United States. It has been mentioned in the literature, but as far as we know, it has not been adopted[a] anywhere in the United States. The author undertook to inquire about this in a nonsystematic way with perhaps 100 or 200 physicians across the country. Some of the comments received follow:

1. A noted physician in private practice in California who had been elected to many national offices in medical professional societies was aware of the Mathur study. However, he said if he took care of an MI (myocardial infarction) patient at home and the patient died, reference to this study and any number of expert witnesses would not serve to convince a California jury that this was not malpractice.
2. A family physician in a small New York town said he has had this article sitting on his desk for two years and knows of

a. McNeer et al.[25] did not even cite the Mathur study.[26]

several patients he would have liked to have cared for at home, but he does not dare attempt it because of the malpractice threat.

3. Two lawyers on the administrative staffs of two hospitals, both with over 600 beds, read the Mathur study and, after a lengthy discussion of it, were asked whether they would prefer to defend a physician whose MI patient died at home or in the hospital. They both thought the hospital death would be an easier case to defend against malpractice.

4. A chief of medicine at a large teaching hospital analyzed the Mathur trial as follows:

Some MI patients in Bristol were not included in the study because their physicians wanted to make the decision whether to treat them at home or in hospital and refused to have them randomized.

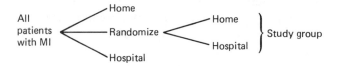

This is true in all clinical trials if, for no other reason, the patient can choose not to be randomized. If one assumes that some patients benefit more from hospitalization and others more from home care, patients could be rank ordered accordingly. If one further assumes that physicians have a high degree of ability to estimate this difference, one could conclude that the patients who were randomized in the Mathur study were preselected to be in the middle range where home and hospital care conferred about the same benefits. This phenomenon is diagrammatically represented in Figure 5.1.

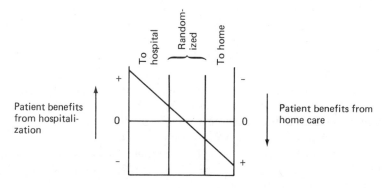

Figure 5-1. Ranking of patients by benefit from hospitalization and by benefit from home care.

Figure 5.1 implies that the randomized group was a group for which the differences in benefits were negligible.

Interesting as this study might be, therefore, it may not help the American clinician because it fails to provide any criteria that will help the clinician place a patient on the scale of benefits and thereby choose appropriate treatment more precisely.

5. America has a vast economic commitment to coronary care units. Physicians concerned with the treatment of MIs are often hospital based, and although very familiar with the Mathur study, they do not feel they are in a position to test it because they have no control over the decision to admit the patient. Furthermore, Bristol, England, has a well-developed home care program; the United States less so. Thus resource shifts would be required here.

We have perhaps digressed too much on this one study, but because it reflects a cluster of issues and because its potential dollar impact is very large, it is as good a case example as can be found.

POSTHOSPITAL AND LONG-TERM CARE

Careful discharge planning has long been known to be effective in reducing hospital use. The elderly patient in need of a nursing home bed is the typical example. Discharge planning is an activity that many hospital nursing and social service departments are well prepared to handle.

Home care is another way to reduce hospital utilization. However, it has its problems. Many hospital-based home care programs in this country are too small. Third-party payers are careful in covering home care to avoid committing themselves to paying for the large numbers of patients who might be involved. One study of home care following hospitalization in New York showed that 40 percent of home care days were substituted for hospital days whereas 60 percent of home care days were in addition to hospital care.[27]

Nursing home care is subject to the same range of variation as is the case for hospital care. If third parties pay liberally for nursing home care, one could imagine that the use of nursing homes would only be limited by the total number of needy elderly persons who are not currently in the hospital. Some observers of the nursing home industry say that a large proportion of these patients would not have to be in nursing homes if alternatives were available. For example, there is a shortage of housing for the elderly. Apartments without flights of stairs, near public transportation, and with access to prepared meals and visiting nurse and social worker programs could reduce the need for nursing home care.

Nursing homes are in part a result of modern industrial society with mobile nuclear families. In an agrarian country like Nigeria nursing homes are unknown. Families are expected to care for their elderly. Surely many a large old New England farmhouse was built with a room for grandmother.

If we wish to cope with the costs of chronic care for the elderly, we may have to address ourselves to a broader social policy. To take one of many questions raised by our social policy: Quite a few elderly retire abroad. A Portugese-American from New Bedford, Massachusetts, may retire to the Azores, while the widow of a physician in Boston spends half her year in a house in Spain. What does this do to the costs of American medical care? At present Massachusetts, under Medicaid, will pay $30 a day for an eligible elderly person in a nursing home. What if the state offered this person's family $25 a day to care for this person at home? How many relatives would accept the state's offer? We do not know.

Psychiatric Hospitalization

As medical historians look back on the last twenty years of medical care, they are likely to say that the most striking event was the massive deinstitutionalization of psychiatric inpatients. The peak U.S. nonfederal psychiatric hospital census was in 1955 when there were 677,000 inpatients. While total hospital expenses grew ninefold from $5.6 billion in 1955 to $48.7 billion in 1975, nonfederal psychiatric hospital total expenses grew only fourfold from $0.9 billion to $4 billion.[17] These figures are summarized in Table 5.5.

This extraordinary transformation has come about as a result of effective psychiatric drugs and the growth of the community mental health movement. Without a doubt, it is one of the most exciting phenomena in medical care.

The number of psychiatric beds varies substantially from one country to another as Table 5.6 shows. In 1969 Sweden had over six times the number of psychiatric beds as the Soviet Union, with America falling in between.

The low number of psychiatric beds in the Soviet Union is an interesting example of how ideology can influence medical care. According to Marxist theory, mental illness is, with a small number of exceptions like tumors and war injury, a result of class conflict. Socialist Russia in abolishing classes, therefore, also abolished class conflict; hence there should be almost no mental illness and little need for psychiatric beds. The Soviet Union frequently has been

Table 5.5. Nonfederal Psychiatric Hospitals in the United States (1955 to 1975), Services and Expenses[17]

	1955	1960	1965	1970	1975
Number of hospitals	542	488	483	519	544
Number of beds (thousands)	707	722	685	527	330
Admissions (thousands)	312	362	419	598	604
Census (thousands)	677	672	607	447	265
Outpatient visits (thousands)	—	—	1003	2740	5287
Total expense (millions)	$923	$1025	$1662	$2712	$3997
Cost per patient day	$3.73	$4.91	$7.50	$16.61	$41.36

Source: American Hospital Association, Hospital Statistics, 1976 Edition, Chicago, 1976. Table 1.

Table 5.6. Psychiatric Beds per 1000 Population by Country, 1969[3]

Sweden	6.28
Ireland	5.7
England and Wales	3.83
Netherlands (1968)	3.22
United States	3.03
France	2.19
Italy	2.16
West Germany	1.89
Portugal	1.03
Soviet Union (1967)	0.97

criticized for committing political dissidents to mental hospitals. One imagines, from the official Kremlin point of view, that any Russian who criticizes the Soviet Union must be a traitor, spy, or crazy.[28,29,30] Some American observers believe there is as much mental illness in the Soviet Union as elsewhere, but Soviet ideology has simply let it go officially unrecognized.

CASE STUDIES TO EXPLAIN VARIATIONS IN INPATIENT CARE

Inguinal Hernia Operations

This, usually elective, procedure is one of the most frequent reasons for hospital admission.[18] Therefore, it can be used as a good example of the issues associated with hospital care and costs.

Bunker observed that twice as many hernia operations per 10,000 population are performed in America as in England and Wales,[31] although no such variation was found in Vermont by Wennberg.[32]

It has long been known that most elective herniorraphies can be done on an outpatient basis for both adults[33,34] and children[35,36] including one randomized trial.[37] Several surgeons have advocated early discharge following surgery.[38,39,40,41] Carroll Bellis reports a series of 11,000 inguinal herniorraphies with immediate unrestricted activity after operation and the use of local anesthesia.[42] There are two randomized trials of home versus hospital care immediately after surgery.[43,44] There is debate over the usefulness of a preoperative barium enema.[45] The benefits of elective herniorraphy in the elderly are debatable.[46] There is substantial variation in length of stay with average stays as high as twelve days being reported in some parts of England in 1960[13] and Scotland in 1967[14] for unobstructed inguinal hernias and hernioplasty.

There appear to be large differences in recurrence rates of hernias after surgery and, therefore, with the costs related to the frequency of repeated surgery.[47,48,49,50,51,52] Toronto's Shouldice Hospital, which specializes in hernia surgery, has a high volume of cases (25,000 patients in fifteen years) and very low mortality and recurrence rates[53,54] (less than 1 percent). Should such specialized high-volume institutions be a model for medical care? Finally, there is Dr. Velez-Gil's remarkable effort to reduce the costs of hernia surgery in Cali, Columbia.[55] Faced with an overwhelming backlog of need, he undertook to lower the costs required by as much as possible consistent with good care. As a result he reduced the cost per case by 75 percent.[55] Perhaps what is remarkable about this study is not the result, but that he did it at all.

This brief summary provides not only answers but is also intended to convey the large range of issues that can be addressed about this frequent surgical procedure. Such an approach could be taken with many other procedures. Which of these cost-saving approaches should be adopted and which rejected? Surely these questions could challenge many an inquiring mind.

The William Douglas Solution

In 1720 the town of Boston had about ten thousand inhabitants and only one physician with a real medical degree, William Douglas, an Edinburgh graduate. The other practitioners had either been trained as apprentices or were clergymen who provided medical care to their parishioners in case of need.

Dr. William Douglas, in a letter to his friend, Dr. Cadwallader

Colden of New York, described how he was paid. This may be the earliest description of medical economics in this country. Douglas writes:

> I have practice amongst four sorts of people: some families pay me five pounds per annum each for advice, sick or well, some few fee me as in Britain, but, for the native New Englanders, I am obliged to keep a day book of my Consultations, Advice and Visits and bring them a bill: others of the poorer sort I advise and visit without any expectation of fees.[56]

"Five pounds per annum each for advice sick or well" is the basic idea behind an HMO; enrolled subscribers and a fixed yearly premium cover a wide range of medical benefits.

"Some few see me as in Britain." To be a British gentleman in the 1700s one could not send a bill for services because that would make one a common merchant. "Bring them a bill" is presumably the current practice among native Americans. "Of the poorer sort I advise and visit without any expectation of fees." Medicare, Medicaid, and government hospitals are, presumably, to make such charity obsolete. However, one doubts that true charity will ever disappear because physicians will always be intellectually challenged by unusual illnesses and devote more time to such patients than their pay would justify in a narrow economic sense.

Let us return to "five pounds per annum, sick or well." By the early part of this century such forms of compensation had gone out of fashion. Here is a quotation from an extraordinary book, *The Physician Himself*, written by Dr. D. W. Cathell in 1922.[57] This book should be read by anyone who believes in the mythical golden age of the old-fashioned family doctor. It was a dog-eat-dog medical world with ill-trained graduates from one of the medical schools closed down by Abraham Flexner on every block in fierce competition one with another. The cut of one's coat, the size of one's horsedrawn carriage, one's bedside manner and the ability to cultivate the well-to-do meant the difference between starvation and affluence. Here is Dr. Cathell's opinion of "five pounds per annum":

> Never enter into an auction bargain to attend an individual or a family, *by the week; month; or year.* It is far better to be paid for what you actually do; than to have part of your patients feel that they are giving you twenty dollars for five dollars' worth of yearly services; while you, on the other hand are; in many other exacting cases, giving fifty or a hundred dollars worth of services for twenty dollars; and have no alternative but to fulfill the Cheap John contract. Avoid all such pitfalls.[57]

Was Dr. Cathell primarily concerned about the "pooling of risks" or the "Cheap John contract" that resulted from auctioning off blocks of patients to the lowest bidder among starving physicians? Not all such contracts had to be like this. There is the tale of the East Coast society doctor thirty years ago who cared for only one hundred families at a set yearly fee of $1000 per family exclusive of hospital expenses, of course. Thirty years ago that was not a "Cheap John contract."[b]

Recent history has led many observers of medical care in the United States to believe that health maintenance organizations are new, very expensive to start, and compete with fee-for-service physicians. This does not necessarily have to be true. The discussion of Mervin Shalowitz's Intergroup Prepaid Health Service in Chapter 6 is interesting because it makes the HMO concept available to small groups of practicing fee-for-service physicians. Intergroup brings the William Douglas solution into the present.

REFERENCES

1. Dumbaugh, Karen. The effects of pre-admission testing on length of stay. *Inquiry*, 13:13–28, Sept. 1976 (Suppl.).
2. Anderson, Odin W. *Health Care: Can There Be Equity?* New York, Wiley, 1972, p. 236.
3. Maxwell, Robert. *Health Care: The Growing Dilemma*, 2nd ed. New York, McKinsey & Co., 1975, p. 27. Soviet Union data for 1967.
4. Simpson, J., et al. *Custom and Practice in Medical Care.* London, Oxford University Press, 1968.
5. Anderson, R., and Hull, J. Hospital utilization and cost trends in Canada and the United States. *Health Serv. Res.*, 4, 3:198–222, fall 1969.
6. Office of Health Economics. *Efficiency in Hospital Service.* London, 1967.
7. For example, Kohn and White. *Health Care.* New York, Oxford University Press, 1977.
8. Greenlick, M. R. The impact of prepaid group practice on American medical care: A critical evaluation. *Ann. Am. Acad. Polit. Soc. Sci.*, pp. 100–113, Jan. 1972.
9. Greenlick, M. R., et al. Comparing the use of medical care services by the medically indigent and a general membership population in a comprehensive prepaid group practice program. *Med. Care*, 10:187–200, May–June 1972.

b. This tale may be the daydreaming of Boston academic physicians who felt they were paid less than their due. This tale was later elaborated. The doctor was said not to have reported this income on his income tax, was caught, convicted, and went to jail.

10. Gaus, Clifton, Cooper, B. S., and Hirschman, C. G. Contrasts in HMO and fee-for-service performance. *Social Security Bull.*, 39, 5:3-14, 1976.
11. Altman, Isidore. Some factors affecting hospital length of stay. *Hospitals JAHA*, 39:68, July 16, 1965.
12. Halter, S. *Factors Affecting the Length of Stay in Hospital.* Strasbourg, Council of Europe, European Public Health Committee, 1968.
13. Heasman, M. A. How long in hospital? *Lancet*, 2:539-541, Sept. 12, 1964.
14. Heasman, M. A., and Carstairs, Vera. Inpatient management: Variations in some aspects of practice in Scotland. *Brit. Med. J.*, 1:495-498, Feb. 27, 1971.
15. Lev, Irving. Day of the week and other variables affecting hospital admissions, discharges and length of stay for patients in the Pittsburgh area. *Inquiry*, 3, 1:3-39, Feb. 1966.
16. McCorkle, L. P. Duration of hospitalization prior to surgery. *Health Serv. Res.*, 5:114-131, Summer 1970.
17. American Hospital Association. *Hospital Statistics*, 1976 ed. Chicago, 1976, Table 1. Published yearly.
18. Commission on Hospital Activities, Ann Arbor, Michigan.
19. Jonsson, Egon, and Neuhauser, D. Hospital staffing ratios in the United States and Sweden. *Inquiry*, 12, 3:128-137, June 1975.
20. Neuhauser, D., and Andersen, R. In Basil Georgopoulos (ed.), *Organizational Research on Health Institutions.* Ann Arbor, Mich.: Institute for Social Research, 1972.
21. Ashley, J. S. A., et al. How much clinical investigation? *Lancet*, 1:890-893, April 22, 1972.
22. Halperin, W., and Neuhauser, D. MEU: A way of measuring efficient utilization of hospital services. *Health Care Manage. Rev.*, 1, 2:63-70, Spring 1976.
23. Varco, Richard L., and Delaney, John (eds.). *Controversy in Surgery.* Philadelphia, W. B. Saunders, 1976.
24. Reid, Duncan, and Barton, T. C. *Controversy in Obstetrics and Gynecology.* Philadelphia, W. B. Saunders, 1969.
25. McNeer, J. Frederick, et al. Hospital discharge one week after acute myocardial infarction. *N. Engl. J. Med.*, 298, 5:229-232, Feb. 2, 1978.
26. Mathur, H. G., et al. Acute myocardial infarction: Home and hospital treatment. *Brit. Med. J.*, 3:334-338, 1971.
27. Associated Hospital Service of New York. *Home Care Following Hospitalization.* New York, 1962.
28. Field, Mark. Psychiatry and ideology: The official Soviet View of Western theories and practices. *Am. J. Psychother.*, 22, 4:602-615, Oct. 1968.
29. Field, Mark. Soviet and American approaches to mental illness. *Rev. Sov. Med. Sci.* (Munch), Nov. 1, 1963.
30. Field, Mark, and Aronson, Jason. The institutional frame-work of Soviet psychiatry. *J. Nerv. Ment. Dis.*, 138:305-322, April 1964.
31. Bunker, John, M.D. Personal communication.
32. Wennberg, Jack. Personal communication.
33. Farquarson, L. Early ambulation with special reference to herniorrhaphy as an outpatient procedure. *Lancet*, 2:517-519, Sept. 10, 1955. Farquarson

reports a series of 485 cases that would have meant the use of 4850 inpatient days surgery was performed under local anesthesia at Royal Infirmary in Edinburgh, Scotland.

34. Rodriguez, Raimundo, and Phillips, John. Inguinal herniorrhaphy as an outpatient procedure. *Int. Surg.* 48, 6:561–565, Dec. 1967.
35. Othersen, H. B., and Clatworthy, H. W. Outpatient herniorrhaphy for infants. *Am. J. Dis. Child.*, 116:78–80, July 1968.
36. Slim, Michel, and Mishalany, Henrig. Outpatient inguinal herniorrhaphy in childhood. *Brit. J. Clin. Pract.*, 25, 5:223–225, May 1971.
37. Shah, C. P., et al. Day care surgery for children. *Med. Care*, 10, 5:437–450, Sept.-Oct. 1972.
38. Chant, A. D. B., et al. Another approach to the hernia waiting list. *Lancet*, 2:1017–1018, Nov. 11, 1972.
39. Doran, F. S. A., et al. The scope and safety of short-stay surgery in the treatment of groin herniae and varicose veins. *Brit. J. Surg.*, 59, 5:333–339, May 1972.
40. Lichtenstein, Irving. Immediate ambulation and return to work following herniorrhaphy. *Indus. Med. Surg.*, pp. 754–759, Sept. 1966.
41. Tetirick, Jack. Early discharge following inguinal herniorrhaphy. *Ohio Med. J.*, 66, 1:41–43, Jan. 1970.
42. Bellis, Carroll. Immediate unrestricted activity after operation. *Int. Surg.*, 55, 4:256–264, April 1971.
43. Echeverri, O., et al. Postoperative care: In hospital or at home? *Int. J. Health Serv.*, 2, 1:101–110, 1972. Patients were randomized and sent home three to five hours after surgery or kept in the hospital, thus reducing the cost to one-fourth of that of hospital care (Tulane University).
44. Morris, David, et al. Early discharge after hernia repair. *Lancet*, 1:681–685, March 30, 1968. Randomized one-day versus six-day postsurgery discharge.
45. Brandel, Thomas, and Kirsch, Israel. Lack of association between inguinal hernia and carcinoma of the colon. *New Engl. J. Med.*, 284:369–370, Feb. 18, 1971.
46. Neuhauser, D., and Gilbert, John. In John Bunker et al. (eds.), *Costs, Risks and Benefits of Surgery*. New York, Oxford University Press, 1977.
47. Blodgitt, James, and Beattie, E. J. The effect of early postoperative rising on the recurrence rate of hernia. *Surg. Gynecol. Obst.*, pp. 716–718, 1947.
48. Quillinan, Robert H. Repair of recurrent inguinal hernia. *Am. J. Surg.*, 118:593–595, Oct. 1969.
49. Thieme, E. Thurston. Recurrent inguinal hernia. *Arch. Surg.*, 103:238–240, Aug. 1971.
50. Postlethwait, R. W. Causes of recurrence after inguinal herniorrhaphy. *Surgery*, 69, 5:772–775, May 1971.
51. Postlethwait, R. W. Recurrent inguinal hernia. *Am. J. Surg.*, 107:739–743, May 1964.
52. Rostad, Hans. Inguinal hernia in adults. *Acta Chird. Scand.*, 134:49–54, 1968.
53. Glassow, Frank. Recurrent inguinal and femoral hernia: 3000 cases. *Can. J. Surg.*, 7:284–288, July 1964.

54. Ues, J. D. H. Specialization in elective herniorrhaphy. *Lancet*, 1:751–755, April 3, 1965.
55. Velez-Gil, Adolfo, et al. A simplified system for surgical operations: The economics of treating hernia. *Surgery*, 77, 3:391–394, March 1975. About half this saving was going from three days in hospital to outpatient surgery, reduced cost of equipment, drugs and supplies, and performing two operations simultaneously in one operating room.
56. Winslow, Ola E. *A Destroying Angel*. Boston, Houghton Mifflin, 1974, pp. 164–189.
57. Cathell, D. W. *Book on the Physician Himself from Graduation to Old Age*. Philadelphia, F. A. Davis, 1931, p. 279.

Chapter 6

Cost Containment
in Inpatient Care

*Mervin Shalowitz**

We are interested in resource management. How efficiently the physician practices and manages limited resources has become a priority topic only recently. This chapter is, therefore, directed toward an explanation of the many forces necessary to change behavior patterns if we are to achieve the most effective use of limited resources and also to realize results desired on behalf of hospitalized patients.

The concept of "cost containment" has often been equated with the rationing of medical care. However, cost effectiveness does not necessarily result in restricting costs or reducing the amount of money spent. It is better equated with the concept of appropriateness of care. Perhaps as physicians, we should not be lured into using the term cost containment or should we be concerned about costs in the sense of containment. Consider instead the physician who wants to practice high-quality medicine, by choosing the most effective therapeutic and diagnostic modalities, by setting sensible levels of care, such as not hospitalizing patients unnecessarily, by prescribing

*Excutive Director, Intergroup Prepaid Health Services, Inc.; Clinical Professor of Medicine, Stritch School of Medicine of Loyola University; Trustee, American Society of Internal Medicine.

The opinions expressed are those of the author and not necessarily those of ASIM or any other organization.

drugs rationally and ordering generic drugs when quality is known, and by using home health care or ambulatory surgery facilities when appropriate. If the physician does all of these things, so-called cost containment will follow naturally as an effect. A motivational concern is necessary to achieve the desired results. Physicians must be willing to assume responsibility for their actions as well as provide the appropriate level of care for each patient. A more appropriate utilization of resources will follow. There must be not only an understanding of but also the capability and willingness to carry out these appropriate procedures.

In discussing cost containment in the inpatient sector from a physician's viewpoint there are four main factors to be considered. First, does the patient need admission? That is, does the patient need the admission to the hospital in the first place or could the necessary services be rendered satisfactorily on an outpatient basis or at a facility offering a less intensive service capability? Second, once the patient is admitted to the hospital, is he or she admitted to the appropriate level of care? That is, is the use of the critical care unit, the coronary care unit, or the intensive care unit necessary, or should the patient be on a surveillance unit or a general floor, or perhaps, if available, a self-care unit? Third, what type of services are ordered for the patient in the hospital? What are the extents of therapy and of testing ordered? And fourth, what are the parameters that determine the length of stay once the patient is admitted to the inpatient facility?

In considering cost containment, we must also consider the reason for cost containment. For whom are we containing costs? This becomes a public problem, particularly when more and more federal money is being spent and when the public is clamoring for more effective use of their money. Not only the patient, but also third-party payers, commercial insurers, Blue Cross–Blue Shield, other fiscal intermediaries, the federal government, employers, and unions are involved and concerned. In other words, the cost containment movement derives from many sources and is primarily important from the standpoint of making maximal use of a finite public resource.

Why has this problem arisen at this time? First, we have strong financial pressures at play with financial incentives skewed toward overspending and overutilization of the existing resources for treatment. For example, we must understand the objectives of the three major parties who are concerned with spending.

We have what I call the party of the first part—the patient. The patient usually has inpatient care covered by some kind of health insurance that the patient either pays for fully or partially, directly or indirectly. Therefore, the patient wants to use this health insurance to be protected against any loss or cost that might be incurred in relation to an illness. Most coverage is hospital coverage, and payment will be made only when the patient is hospitalized. Thus patients exert pressure on the system to utilize this level of care for any medical service rendered to them for an intercurrent illness or injury. Of course, patients also have a preconceived idea that a higher quality of care may be rendered in a hospital as compared to care provided in am ambulatory setting.

Next we have the party of the second part—the physician. Physicians see the patient with a hospitalization policy as a guarantee toward payment for their services and for all other services that will be rendered on behalf of the patient. In addition, physicians see the hospital as a convenient location for taking care of the patient, particularly physicians who do not have laboratory or x-ray facilities in their office and who know that they can see a larger number of patients in less time and with less bother in the hospital than on an outpatient basis.

We must also admit at this point that physicians have a reimbursement incentive to see patients in a higher cost setting because this is usually where they can also receive a higher compensation for their services.

Finally, we have the party of the third part—the third-party payers. They include the insurance companies, which are no more than fiscal intermediaries, the government, now is responsible for paying up to 40 percent of the health care dollar nationally, and others, such as employers or unions. All are interested in proper utilization of hospitals and hospital resources and, as responsible fiscal intermediaries, are looking for more appropriate expenditures of the health care dollar. But these payers incur the wrath of the parties of the first and second parts if payment is attenuated or denied.

Until recently much of the thrust of organized medicine has been to establish cost with the third-party payers—with Blue Cross–Blue Shield, commercial insurance companies, and the government— to protect the physician and to assure payment of charges, often without any consideration of appropriateness of these charges or the appropriateness of the care rendered to the patient. This, of course, has changed as you can see from Dr. Sammon's statement as well as from the current impact of many major specialty societies, including the American Society of Internal Medicine, in establishing study groups on cost containment.

On August 5, 1977, a task force on cost containment was convened by the American Society of Internal Medicine. The purpose was "To develop recommendations for specific actions to contain the costs of medical care, yet to permit continued improvement of quality." The task force further stated, "Activity should include (a) the economic impact of clinical decision making; (b) HSA's and PSRO's; and (c) changing the attitude (logic and scarcity) and behavior of the clinician." This committee recognized four major categories among which to divide its cost containment ideas. They are (1) cost containment in the hospital setting; (2) cost containment in the office setting; (3) cost containment in relation to the patient; and (4) cost containment in relation to third-party insurance carriers. It has identified a number of problems in these four areas, and its future task will be to determine ways in which to solve these problems.

BACKGROUND

Many of the cost containment ideas that I will discuss have been identified as a result of my activities in the development and operation of a prepaid health plan operating in northern Illinois and adjacent northwestern Indiana, which has been operational since January 1972. At that time, after completing an eighteen-month feasibility study, physicians in private fee-for-service group practices helped form the entity known as Intergroup Prepaid Health Services and contracted with Intergroup to convert part of their fee-for-service practices to a prepayment format. These medical groups provide medical care full-time and have laboratory and x-ray facilities available on site. The medical groups we have under contract are both free-standing and hospital based.

Intergroup is a full-service health plan providing inpatient and outpatient benefits of a comprehensive nature, including out-of-area care and catastrophic coverage for a single premium. Intergroup provides the administrative systems, marketing, actuarial services, and legal services for the group medical practices involved in an areawide prepaid plan. In April 1977 Intergroup became a federally qualified HMO under Title XIII of the Public Health Service Act. As in all prepaid plans, the financial incentive is shifted from the fee-for-service and indemnity system of insurance, with no apparent constraint on funding, to prepayment, which limits funding to a defined budget. Again, I would like to stress that this should not be considered as rationing the health care dollar but merely offering the physician a different form of incentive in allocating the health care dollar.

The Intergroup Plan provides standard comprehensive medical and surgical services to individuals. The physicians in the medical groups receive a monthly capitation fee to provide care for enrollees registered at their particular medical facility. Members are entitled to services on demand without proof of illness, including laboratory and x-ray services on an ambulatory basis as well as treatment for acute and chronic illnesses and periodic physical examinations. The plan includes such services as well-baby care, immunization programs, preschool examinations, and eye examinations. Furthermore, prescription drugs prescribed by participating physicians are included in the capitation premium. Hospitalization benefits are provided, and extended care facility confinement is possible with or without prior hospitalization, as are home health care services. Since the revenue is derived from capitation payments and not from fee-for-service income, the generation of revenue is disengaged from the utilization of medical services. In addition, the physicians have an opportunity through a shared risk fund to utilize premium dollars that may be saved by not using hospitals unnecessarily to expand ambulatory care funding.

It has long been recognized, and has been proven by recent utilization studies, that many hospitalizations are medically unnecessary and that the level of care, extent of services, and lengths of stay often may be inappropriate to the care of the patient. In one study by Dickson and Laszlo,[1] utilization of clinical chemistry services by the medical house staff was analyzed. During the study they concluded that "The percentage of laboratory data that is actually used in diagnosis and treatment of patients is low (5 percent). This percentage can be significantly increased when greater selectivity is required prior to ordering blood chemistry tests." In addition, our experience has borne out the fact that hospitalization days per thousand people can be greatly reduced when the reimbursement incentives are changed. For example, we have found that for our entire plan in 1975 with some 18,000 enrollees, our bed days per thousand were 527 as compared to between 900 and 1100 bed days per thousand for the comparable indemnity experience in the Chicago area. More specifically (Table 6.1), we can see a great savings in hospital bed days in two large enrolled groups of employed people in our program.

So far we have been dealing with physician responsibility in regard to innovations and cost effectiveness. I should now like to speak briefly about the hospital's responsibility in regard to cost effectiveness and particularly in regard to cost containment per se. Table 6.2 shows the daily room and board charges for semiprivate

Table 6.1. Hospital Days per 1000 Members per Year, Intergroup and Blue Cross Enrollees for Two Large Chicago Employers, 1975

	Blue Cross	Intergroup (Prepaid Plan)
Illinois Bell Telephone Co.	983	515
Continental Insurance Co.	918	269

Table 6.2. Hospital Charges for Hospitals Commonly Used by Intergroup

| Hospital | Per Diem Daily Room and Board Charges for: | |
	Semiprivate	ICU
Michael Reese Hospital	$194	$350
Skokie Valley Hospital	121	220
Presbyterian–St. Luke's Hospital	196	349
Central DuPage Hospital	102	190
Palos Community Hospital	112	240
Bethesda Hospital	125	220
Ravenswood Hospital	125	210
Illinois Masonic Hospital	175	320
Mt. Sinai Hospital	150	300
St. Bernard's Hospital	130	225
Roseland Hospital	120	225
Henrotin Hospital	122	275
St. Margaret's Hospital (Hammond)	106	225
St. Francis Hospital (Peoria)	83	90
Burnham Hospital (Champaign)	82	160[a]
Grant Hospital	137	310
Columbus Hospital	131	253–293
Ingalls Hospital	105	200
Lutheran General Hospital	172	199[b]
St. Francis Hospital (Evanston)	115	250
Thorek Hospital	135	200
Tabernacle Hospital	130	No ICU
Mercy Hospital	150	300

[a]Plus hourly charge of $5.00.
[b]Plus $111 for monitoring.

facilities and for the intensive care units in hospitals most commonly used by our prepaid plan. There is a great variation between hospitals in the Chicago area and hospitals located outside of the Chicago area, particularly downstate Illinois. One must wonder to what extent differences in the cost effectiveness of management underlies the wide spread in these daily rates.

While discussing hospitals, I would also like to comment on President Carter's proposed 9 percent gap on annual rises in hospital costs. In my opinion this is a ridiculous proposal. For example, I would like to show how far on or off the 9 percent target a number of representative hospitals are in the Chicago area. Table 6.3 is excerpted from a *Chicago Sun Times* survey published recently. Of the nineteen hospitals surveyed, only one—Skokie Valley Community Hospital— and I have had nothing to do with the survey but it happens to be a hospital in which I practice—has kept all its room rate increases under 9 percent during the past year. The percentages of increase at the other hospitals were generally in the teens and some rose much higher.

We recognize that new technology has a great impact upon the health care costs. However, one cost containment idea that I would like to propose is that papers about new procedures and treatments should be published only with full descriptions of appropriate applications and expected health benefits and only if cost implications are fully described. Discussion should include expected effects on the system as a whole as well as on individual patient care, the locus of treatment, the extent of treatment, and length of stay.

SECOND-OPINION SURGERY

Recently I have been helping design and implement a second-opinion surgery program for a union pension trust that is self-insured and self-administered in the Chicago area. This program began May 1, 1977, and the accumulated experience is tabulated through August 30. There were forty requests for second-opinion elective surgery, and six cases were not confirmed for surgery on the second opinion. Of these cases one operation was performed. Ten members of the union had elective surgery without a second opinion. These data are very preliminary but do suggest a trend and a possible means to obviate some unnecessary elective surgery. The program was developed as a mandatory one in which no payment would be made for elective surgery without a second opinion from a panel of predetermined practitioners in the field in which the surgery was to be performed.

Table 6.3.   Room Rate Increases for Selected Chicago-area Hospitals, 1976–1977

Hospital	1976 Daily Rate	1977 Daily Rate	Percent Increase
Augustana			
Semiprivate	$122	$141.50	16
Private	$135	$158	17
Intensive care	$275	$412.50	50
Louise Burg			
Semiprivate	$45.50	$56.50	24
Private	$46.50	$57.50	24
Intensive care	$55.25	$66.50	20
Children's Memorial			
Semiprivate	$160	$195	22
Private	$170	$205	21
Intensive care	$250	$375	50
Columbus			
Semiprivate	$115	$131	14
Private	$125	$141	13
Intensive care	$230	$253	10
County			
Per-diem rate			
(All services)	$270	$310	15
Grant			
Semiprivate	$122	$137	12
Private	$135	$151	12
Intensive care	$250	$310	24
Hines Veterans			
Per-diem rate			
(All services)	$116.87	$134.74	15
Ingalls			
Semiprivate	$87	$102	17
Private	$92	$107	16
Intensive care	$160	$200	25
Jackson Park			
Semiprivate	$121	$151	25
Private	$139	$174	25
Intensive care	$225	$400	78
Loyola			
Semiprivate	$140	$165	18
Private	$150	$175	17
Intensive care	$310	$335	8
MacNeal Memorial			
Semiprivate	$104	$115	11
Private	$109	$120	10
Intensive care	$225	$250	11

Table 6.3 *(continued)*

Hospital	1976 Daily Rate	1977 Daily Rate	Percent Increase
McHenry			
Semiprivate	$80	$90	13
Private	$92	$102	11
Intensive care	$160	$170	6
Northwestern Mem.			
Semiprivate	$130	$173	33
Private	$151	$179	19
Intensive care	$311	$341	10
Pres-St. Luke's			
Semiprivate	$147	$184	25
Private	$153	$190	24
Intensive care	$300	$337	12
Ravenswood			
Semiprivate	$102	$125	23
Private	$112	$135	21
Intensive care	$185	$210	14
Michael Reese			
Semiprivate	$164	$182	11
Private	$176	$194	10
Intensive care	$320	$350	9
St. Joseph			
Semiprivate	$112	$129	15
Private	$122	$139	14
Intensive care	$170–	$200–	18–
	$215	$300	40
St. Francis			
Semiprivate	$105	$115	10
Private	$107	$120	12
Intensive care	$225	$250	11
Skokie Valley			
Semiprivate	$114	$121	6
Private	$120	$127	6
Intensive care	$205	$220	7

Source: Bob Olmstead, Area hospitals miss 9% target, copyright © 1977, *Chicago Sun-Times.*

Note: Only one of these hospitals, Skokie Valley Community Hospital, kept all its room-rate increases under 9 percent in 1976–1977. As can be seen from the table, other hospitals' percentages of increase were much higher—often in the teens. Also, the *Sun-Times* indicated that "if Carter wants to keep medical costs below a 9-percent yearly rise, he might look first at government-run hospitals." For example, at Hines Veterans Hospital, the per-diem rate rose 15 percent from 1976 to 1977.

However, a negative opinion about proceeding with the surgery would not prevent the procedure from being done if the patient's physician decided to proceed.

It is my opinion that perhaps the second opinion might better be obtained from other specialists than those involved in performing the procedure in question. For example, in considering coronary bypass surgery, we might want to have the opinion of a medical cardiologist rather than a cardiovascular surgeon. Similarly, for lumbar disc disease, it may be advantageous to have the opinion of a neurologist rather than another orthopedic surgeon. Certainly, surgical specialists are more inclined to operate than nonsurgical specialists.

PREADMISSION TESTING

For further cost containment efforts in our prepayment program, we have noted a number of things of general interest. First, routine admission profiles and standing orders, particularly routine postoperative orders by surgeons and standing orders in critical care units or so-called critical care profiles, should be abolished. Orders should be written specifically and tailored to the needs of the patient and the problems in question. To practice cost-effective care, we have found it necessary to negate standing orders, particularly when preadmission testing is done.

On the other hand, preadmission testing, especially for all non-emergent admissions, is not only desirable but also mandatory if we are going to practice cost-effective care. Particularly in elective pre-operative situations, testing should be done before the patient is admitted to the hospital. Furthermore, we should try to convince hospitals to accept preadmission testing done at a locus other than the hospital. Many hospitals currently are unwilling to do this. If the laboratory and x-ray testing is done in a facility with adequate quality assurance procedures and competent personnel and supervision, there is no reason why these test results should not be accepted in any hospital for inclusion on its records. The responsibility for the tests, as well as their interpretation and utilization, still belongs to the attending physician who has been granted staff privileges at the hospital.

GLOBAL FEES

In a recent major publication on cost containment,[2] the authors felt that major changes will not come about quickly or uniformly. They, therefore, produced a document that "sought the middle ground"—cost control activities with the highest potential compatible with conventional medical, hospital, and insurance schemes. I feel that we can go a few steps further and deviate from conventional schemes. Medical fees may be uncoupled from inpatient utilization considerations by using a prepayment plan in the fee-for-service sector in the form of global fees. These global fees are predetermined for total care of a specific problem or diagnosis. We did have such fees in surgical and obstetrical settings until several years ago. This idea should be resurrected and also be applied to medical conditions.

UTILIZATION REVIEW

Control of cost and cost-effective care has to be tied to some kind of a review mechanism. In our program we provide utilization information to our participating physicians with monthly computer printouts that show incurred dollar costs by case. We also provide utilization information to our participating physicians with monthly computer printouts that show incurred dollar cost, hospital admissions and bed days, and frequency and type of ambulatory care visits. The latter data are only now being generated with implementation of an encounter from listing type and site of care. This feedback mechanism also could be implemented in the fee-for-service sector.

CONCLUSIONS AND RECOMMENDATIONS

Based on our experiences and those of others, what are some of the things we can do to increase the awareness of our so-called cost problem?

1. *The Patient.* The patient should receive a copy of itemized charges for all services received together with intelligible identification of those services. This would increase awareness of cost and also would allow the patient to check to be sure that all services were actually rendered. Our experience is such that hospital billing services range from the ridiculous to the superb. We have found many instances of overcharging and mischarging in the way of charges billed to the wrong patient on many hospital bills. The public as patients also should have periodic reminders, preferably through their employers, unions, or even their insurance companies to instruct them how to use their insurance benefits. These notices should be written in

simple language and should state clearly the limitations and responsibility for payment of incurred charges. Patients should also be instructed about how to shop for medical services and should be encouraged to ask about the type of care they are to receive, why it is necessary, and what are the alternatives to treatment. The costs of such services—both the direct and indirect cost—should be known before patients agree to any non-emergent care.

2. *The Physician.* Each staff physician should be provided with a printout of hospital utilization by the physician. The services provided, the cost for each service such as laboratory examinations, x rays, pharmacy, or surgery, as well as the bed days used per case and the cost of the level of care prescribed should all be itemized. They should be correlated with norms established for the diagnosis and for complications experienced, if any, of patients similarly treated.

3. *The Hospital.* The hospital should be encouraged to provide the above information routinely despite the expense of doing so. Hospitals must assume responsibility for cost containment not only through effective management but also by attempting to limit utilization of services that are not necessary from a medical standpoint. It is obvious from Table 6.2 listing the comparative costs of sample hospitals in the Chicago area that many hospitals do not need all of the services they have available. There must be public accountability for hospital operational costs and cost accounting. There must be a guarantee of appropriate utilization of facilities and services. Although this last factor is largely a medical staff function, the successful achievement of objectives is the hospital's responsibility and ultimately rests with the board of trustees of the hospital. In my experience, effective peer review and utilization review do not exist in the indemnity sector. We have had cases referred to hospital utilization and audit committees and also to county medical societies for review, and invariably, they are whitewashed with the phrase, "The physician felt what he did was best for the patient at that time." Somehow hospitals must be encouraged to implement effective length of stay or utilization committees. One need is for scientifically determined criteria to indicate when a patient can safely leave the hospital or be transferred to another, less costly level of care. For example, length of stay for an acute myocardial infarction went from six weeks flat in bed twenty-five years ago to the use of early ambulation now and a nine- to fifteen-day length of stay in

many institutions for acute uncomplicated myocardial infarctions. Other, similar case studies are necessary.

Earlier we discussed preadmission testing as a means of shortening hospital stays. As a variation, the Kaiser Program in Southern California has implemented the policy of admitting patients on the morning of surgery rather than the night before to eliminate an extra overnight bed stay. For nonemergent surgical cases, this is an interesting concept that deserves further consideration.

Finally, the hospitals should be encouraged to facilitate discharge planning. Discharge planning should start with the admission to the hospital. All too often this phase of hospital care can be inadequate or delayed and, therefore, results in unnecessarily long hospitalizations that could have been obviated by earlier identification of the patient's long-term needs for care.

4. *The Third Party.* Insurance companies, Blue Cross–Blue Shield, government employers, and union pension trusts all should be encouraged to:
   a. Write contracts in simple English.
   b. Emphasize exclusions in the contract.
   c. Build in cost-effective language for claims review as well as for promoting responsibility for appropriateness of care to the practicing physician.

There has been a particular reluctance by all the third parties mentioned to become involved in innovations or changes in the patterns of what they perceive as the correct way to receive, provide, or reimburse patients for medical services. These traditions must be breached and new methodologies developed to assure not only continued excellence in the delivery of medical services but also appropriateness for the cost effectiveness of care.

REFERENCES

1. Dixon, R. H., and Laszlo, J. Utilization of clinical chemistry services by medical house staff: An analysis. *Arch. Int. Med.*, 134:1064–1067, Dec. 1974.
2. Griffith, J. R., Hancock, W. M., and Munson, F. C. *Cost Control in Hospitals.* Ann Arbor, Health Administration Press, 1976.

Chapter 7

Peer Evaluation

H. Thomas Ballantine*

In the last few years the average practicing physician has been confronted with a bewildering array of words, phrases, acronyms, and abbreviations that seldom, if ever, were encountered either during medical school or postgraduate training. For example: Peer review, peer evaluation, medical audit, and MCEs, which is an abbreviation for medical care evaluation studies, and to some is slightly more palatable than the term medical audit even though it means the same thing. If this array of terms were not enough, we also have PSRO, FMC, HMO, IPA, and others. At the same time advances in medical technology have all but overwhelmed physicians with the need to upgrade continually their medical knowledge. Is it unusual, then, that the busy physician, whether a general practitioner or neurosurgeon, plaintively asks, "How do I get to my patient's bedside and when will someone give me time to see something of my family?" And is it any wonder that the costs of medical care have, at least until recently, been a low priority item on the list of the practicing physician's concerns?

Nevertheless, the overwhelming majority of physicians in America

*President, Commonwealth Institute of Medicine, Boston.

cling firmly to the belief that the best medical care is rendered in a setting in which an individual physician can enter into an agreement with an individual patient and undertake to treat that patient to the best of his or her ability with the exercise of independent unfettered judgment.

Finally, those who pay for the delivery of medical care are increasingly demanding that "something" be done to control the cost of medical care.

In essence, then, one can identify six essential ingredients that are involved in today's medical care delivery system:

1. Quality
2. Availability
3. Acceptability (of the system to patient and physician alike)
4. Cost
5. Organization
6. Control

Patients, physicians, payers, and politicians give differing priorities to these basic elements as they address them; but as I see the situation, the physician, if he or she wishes to retain some degree of independence as a practitioner and decision maker, must become involved in attempting to solve the problems residing, not in just one or two, but in all six of these fundamental aspects of the delivery of medical care. This can best be accomplished by an understanding of and involvement in the process of peer evaluation and the application of peer influence. One can place this complicated subject in proper perspective by briefly reviewing some aspects of the past, methods of peer evaluation now in use, problem areas uncovered by research, and suggested ways peer evaluation can help reduce costs and improve quality.

PEER EVALUATION DEFINED

Peer evaluation and peer review can be used interchangeably and defined as follows: "Peer Review is the evaluation by practicing physicians of the quality and efficiency of services ordered or performed by other physicians. Peer Review is the all inclusive term for medical review efforts, including medical practice analysis, inpatient hospital and extended care facility utilization review, medical audit, ambulatory care review and claims review."[1]

HISTORICAL ANTECEDENTS TO
PEER EVALUATION

The true birth of the peer review concept occurred shortly after the publication of the Flexner study of medical education in 1910. A group of surgeons who were precursors to the American College of Surgeons was formed. Their initial thrust was to determine the quality of care rendered by reviewing outpatient outcomes in hospital surgical cases. It was physicians, therefore, not the public or the government who took the first steps toward quality assurance and peer evaluation in this country. A central figure in this movement was Earnest Amory Codman (1869–1940), a surgeon at the Massachusetts General Hospital whose pioneer efforts will be described in some detail here.

In 1934, Dr. Codman's classic text, "The Shoulder: Rupture of the Supraspinatus Tendon and Other Lesions In or About the Subacromial Bursa,"[2] was published. In the preface to this volume he recorded in autobiographical fashion his experiences with peer evaluation:

> Already in 1900 I had become interested in what I have called the End Result Idea, which was merely the common-sense notion that every hospital should follow every patient it treats long enough to determine whether or not the treatment has been successful, and then to inquire "if not, why not?" with a view to preventing similar failures in the future. . . . this routine tracing of every case, interesting or uninteresting, had brought to our notice many things in which our knowledge, our technique, our organization, our own skill or wisdom, and perhaps even our care and our consciences, needed attention. . . .

He reviewed the end results of about 600 cases in the previous ten years. He tabulated these cases, not only according to the lesions, but also according to the results of each individual operator. The tables he developed offered overwhelming evidence that good results had not always been obtained by the eighteen (operating) surgeons.

Young Dr. Codman's "End Result Idea" was not looked upon with universal enthusiasm by his colleagues, particularly the senior members of the surgical staff of the Massachusetts General Hospital. He wrote:

> In order to attract the attention of the trustees of the MGH, I resigned from the staff in 1914 "as a protest against the seniority system of promo-

tion," which was obviously incompatible with the End Result Idea. On the day on which I received the acceptance of my resignation, I wrote again, asking to be appointed Surgeon-in-Chief on the ground that the results of my treatment of patients at their (the trustees) hospital during the last ten years, had been better than those of other surgeons. I had tabulated my results in case they should ask to see them, but as no one had ever inquired into the results of other surgeons, there was of course nothing with which to compare mine. Thus, as I had planned, this fact was brought to the notice of the trustees, although at some personal sacrifice on my part.

He arranged a local medical society meeting (of which he was the chairman) on January 6, 1915. He expressed concern that attention was being paid to hospital cleanliness, architecture, and kindliness of the nursing staff, but little attention was directed at whether the treatment was efficient or as successful as possible.

Hospitals then apparently had no one responsible for the results of treatment, much less comparing outcomes of different staff members or making collective comparisons between hospitals of the results attained by the staff as a whole. Efficiency and effectiveness were left to the skills and integrity of the physicians on the staff.

Codman further expressed concern that if the services of one surgeon or physician were different from another, this difference must be capable of demonstration by a comparative test instead of only on the basis of seniority. He was convinced that no physician or surgeon could be expected to be proficient in all branches of a single specialty.

He continues:

> Is it possible to compare therapeutic results in medicine and surgery, or must we admit that no matter how much we read, study, practice and take pains, when it comes to a showdown of the results of our treatment, no one could tell the difference between what we have accomplished and the results of some genial charlatan or some less painstaking and energetic colleague?
>
> Comparisons are odious, but comparison is necessary in science. Until we freely make therapeutic comparisons, we cannot claim that a given hospital is efficient, for efficiency implies that the results have been looked into. Hospital efficiency is mainly therapeutic efficiency.

These efforts to promote outcome studies were indeed "odious" to Codman's peers. He was never reappointed to the active staff of the Massachusetts General Hospital following his resignation in 1914 despite the fact that his End Result Idea continues to operate to this day at the Massachusetts General.

Codman's contribution has almost been forgotten, and peer evaluation is thought by some to be something totally new. Moreover, the idea of comparing the quality of care and "efficiency" of one practitioner with another has never been popular. Indeed, in England in which the National Health Service is thought by some to be a model for changes in our own system, peer review is felt by most British physicians to be an intolerable intrusion into the patient-physician relationship!

METHODS OF PEER EVALUATION

Since the early efforts of Codman and the American College of Surgeons, a number of approaches to peer review and quality assurance have been developed. A small sample of these methods will be discussed briefly here.

The American Medical Association[3] published a peer review manual that described eight steps to be undertaken in conducting peer review along with specific advice regarding approaches to utilization review, medical audit, ambulatory care review, and claims review. Williamson has proposed a structured method quality assurance involving (1) selection of priority teams, (2) training sessions, (3) incubation, (4) priority-setting meetings, and (5) selection of topics for implementation. He maintains that only in this manner (using multidisciplinary teams that encourage nonphysician input) can a more holistic view of health care improvement be undertaken.[4] Brown conceived the bi-cycle concept, which relates the patient care cycle to the continuing medical education cycle. A gap between the actual practice and the criteria represents the improvement potential. Closing the gap by directly incorporating materials into the educational program objective is a major function of peer evaluation in this concept.[5] Others have researched the effects of different kinds of peer evaluation on types of problems uncovered. Results here indicate that different methods will produce substantially different results when measuring quality of care. The most valid approach to assessing the quality of care, given the present state of the art, is individual case analysis of both medical care process and patient outcome. Interestingly, the least effective method apeared to be measuring the quality of care rendered against a list of process criteria.[6,7] Others looking at quality of care in hospitals suggested the on-site audit as the best method to maintain high standards of practice within a hospital.[8] Browning, on the other hand, suggests that using hospital records alone is too limited for conducting quality assurance programs.[9]

Mitchell suggests three basic methods of conducting peer evaluation:

1. Compare each physician with his or her peer.
2. Provide educational feedback to physicians about their practice patterns.
3. Surveillance—watch over the kinds of services rendered by practitioners in different settings. By anticipating the need to have some peer evaluation efforts impact on health care costs, Mitchell suggests that hospitals could require written preoperative reports from attending physicians; require written pre- and postoperative consultations; and restrict hospital privileges for selected types of procedures.[10]

LEGISLATION OF UTILIZATION REVIEW AND PSRO

Peer evauation received its first formal endorsement with the enactment of the Medicare and Medicaid amendments in 1965. Congress was properly concerned at that time over the possibility that increased access to medical care by the poor and the elderly could lead to inappropriate utilization of acute hospital facilities. Hospitals were, therefore, required to appoint and staff utilization review committees, whose task was to monitor the use of hospital services, including length of stay, by Medicare and Medicaid patients. Although a certain pious statement about "quality" was put forth, the main thrust of this in-hospital committee approach was to attempt to eliminate, or at least to reduce, overutilization of services.

As has been adequately documented again and again, this approach was less than satisfactory. Hospitals with high occupancy rates had efficient utilization review committees and those whose occupancy rates were low had inefficient, lackadaisical committees. Moreover, little or no attempt was made to monitor in-hospital ancillary services as to their appropriateness and necessity.

Congress and the American taxpayers were alarmed at the rapidly escalating expenditures for Medicare and Medicaid brought about by a combination of inflation, better wages for hospital workers, overutilization of services, and inefficient in-hospital practices. The product of this consternation and frantic search for solutions was the passage of the so called Bennett Amendment (PL 92–603) in October of 1972—an act that created Professional Standards Review Organizations commonly (but not necessarily affectionately) referred to as PSROs. This legislation mandated the creation of PSRO areas throughout the nation, and currently there are 195.

Although the expressed intent of the legislation was to improve the quality and "efficiency" (to use Codman's term) of the care of Medicaid and Medicare patients, it was felt by its sponsors that these efforts would inevitably impact favorably on the costs of medical care. Many practitioners, however, expressed the view that the PSRO legislation would lower the quality of medical care by placing intolerable restrictions on the judgment of physicians, leading to something called "cookbook medicine," reduction in the provision of needed services to patients, and unwarranted intrusion into the patient-physician relationship. Review of an innovative Massachusetts program will serve as a review of what has happened since the passage of PSRO.

PEER EVALUATION EFFORTS IN
MASSACHUSETTS

During the period of 1965 to 1970, the Massachusetts Medical Society became increasingly concerned with the impact of socioeconomic problems on the practice of medicine. This concern led to the formation in 1972 of the Commonwealth Institute of Medicine (CIM), an independent nonprofit corporation whose bylaws require on its board of twenty-one members, representation from practicing physicians, Blue Cross, Blue Shield, The Health Insurance Association of America, The Massachusetts Hospital Association, labor, the consumer, and the state and federal governments.

The state launched two peer evaluation efforts that will be described in detail: one, concurrent monitoring of acute in-hospital care with primary emphasis on utilization of hospital beds was sponsored and supported by the government. The other focused primarily on the activities of physicians in and out of the hospital. This was supported by the private sector.

Early in 1973 the Department of Public Welfare of the Commonwealth of Massachusetts found itself in danger of losing its Medicaid subsidy from the federal government because of a lack of a satisfactory program for utilization review of Medicaid beneficiaries in acute hospitals. Five PSRO areas had been designated in Massachusetts, but the PSROs themselves had not yet been formed.

After lengthy negotiations, the Department of Public Welfare entered into a contract with CIM to implement the Commonwealth Hospital Admissions Monitoring Program (CHAMP). At that time the final regulations for PSRO activity .had not been issued, but the CHAMP contract was written to conform to the PSRO legislation and designed to allow the review process to be a "pre-view of PSRO."

CHAMP became operational in October of 1973 and terminated in August of 1977 when the PSROs implemented formal review of Medicaid patients. The program operated as follows: allied health professionals, employed as utilization review coordinators by CIM, monitored admissions of Medicaid (Title XIX) patients in 125 acute hospitals. Length of stay was monitored concurrently by using the 50th and 75th percentiles of Professional Activities Study Length of Stay norms for the northeastern United States as of 1971. As the 50th percentile date approached and it was obvious that an additional length of stay was indicated, the coordinator could independently extend to the 75th percentile. If the coordinator could not find a reason for extension or if the patient remained in the hospital up to the 75th percentile, consultation with a hospital-based physician advisor was required. If the physician advisor could not justify a length of stay after consultation with the patient's physician, payment to the hospital was denied. An appeal from this decision could be made to a local committee formed by a foundation for medical care in the hospital's geographic area. An adverse decision from this committee could be appealed to the CHAMP State Committee. This latter group not only heard appeals but also set policy for the administration of the CHAMP program. The committee was composed of five representatives from the five Foundations for Medical Care in Massachusetts, two representatives from the Massachusetts Hospital Association, four consumer representatives, and two officers from the Commonwealth Institute of Medicine.

During the period October 1973 to August 1977 approximately 350,000 admissions of Medicaid patients to the 125 acute hospitals were monitored. It is of interest that in only sixteen instances were there appeals to local committees, and in no instance was an appeal carried to the CHAMP State Committee. Of these appeals, six decisions upheld the adverse finding of the physician advisor, and in ten cases the decision was overturned.

A study of the impact of this program on utilization rates showed that the average length of stay of Medicaid patients was reduced by 5.3 percent, compared to non-Medicaid patients. During this four-year period the reductions represented a gross savings to the Commonwealth of $22 million and a net savings of $16.5 million in hospital charges.

The impact of the quality assurance program on the medical care rendered in Massachusetts is more difficult to evaluate. There were, however, three instances in which hospitals were disciplined. Investigation of two of these hospitals disclosed inappropriate and unnecessary hospital stays and surgery. The third hospital was found to be charging for acute hospital stay while acting primarily as an alcoholic detoxification center.

The surgeons in the hospitals rendering inappropriate care were also disciplined, and one has appeared before the Board of Registration and Discipline in Medicine for possible revocation of his license.

The CHAMP program also increased physician awareness of the need to expand Codman's in-hospital concept of peer evaluation to a statewide peer review activity and made it possible for Blue Shield of Massachusetts to expand its own program of utilization review.

In 1973 Blue Shield entered into a series of contracts with the Foundations for Medical Care in Massachusetts (whose territorial boundaries coincide with those of the PSROs) to undertake utilization review of physicians' services at a local level. The following is an overview of the program: staff nurses at Blue Shield headquarters review claims chosen from four principal sources, prepayment screens, computerized norms, random sampling, and complaints from physicians, hospitals, other providers, and thid party payers. If the appropriateness of payment is questioned at this level, a "level II" review is instituted, involving consultation by the nurses with on-site physician reviewers provided by the foundations. If this second review process is reaffirmed, a "level III" review is implemented. This review of the most difficult problems is undertaken by an ad hoc panel of at least three specialists in the particular medical discipline in question. Such a review may also be requested by any physician who feels aggrieved by a level I or a level II decision.

The latest report of three years of operation disclosed that more than $20 million has been saved or recovered by this type of peer evaluation. For every dollar spent by Blue Shield on utilization review more than $6 has been returned to the corporation. The number of physicians impacted adversely by this activity is minimal; Blue Shield deals with some 20,000 health care providers in all fields, and the estimated $8 million recovered in 1977 is only about 4 percent of a projected $205 million in total claims incurred. Nevertheless, in the past three years seventy-five physicians have had formal review of their activities and fifty-one have been disciplined, some for the rendering of care that was completely unnecessary or inappropriate.

Although reduction in length of stay for Medicaid patients was more dramatic, there was an overall reduction in length of stay for all

patients. This suggests that this form of peer evaluation in Massachusetts has been demonstrated to be a cost-effective mechanism that
can also improve the quality of patient care. Moreover, timely
application of this approach to the private sector as well as to the
PSRO programs offers the best chance for preventing a headlong
plunge into a national health service with its potential disatrous
shortcomings.

The programs described have been cost effective primarily by
trimming the inefficiencies within the system. They were both also
achieved by absolute private sector involvement. If, however, peer
evaluation in all its aspects is undertaken with careful regard to the
principles of Codman, then certainly we will discover underutiliza-
tion as well as overutilization, that appropriate procedures are sometimes inappropriately omitted, and that the fat we trim may not
compensate in dollars for the increased cost of rendering high-quality
care.

I do not fear this possibility. There is no reason why 8.6 percent
or 9 percent or 10 percent of the gross national product is too much
to spend for medical care so long as approximately $2 billion is being
spent on bubble gum! I believe that the public is willing to support a
costly medical care delivery system of high quality if that system has
programs for clear accountability and assurance to the individual
who ultimately pays the bill that he or she has received a benefit at
least equal to the cost of the service.

ISSUES IN PEER EVALUATION

While these peer evaluation programs in Massachusetts appear
to have achieved considerable successes, nationwide, many issues remain to be resolved. Research on methods to effect improvements in
peer review and research aimed to explicate existing inefficiencies in
the health care system provide ample fodder for consideration. The
following list will provide some examples:

1. The average level of patient care does not necessarily improve
   when increased time is allocated to direct patient care.[11]
2. Quantity, quality, and cost of medical care in the United States
   is not always the best.
3. Patients with psychiatric symptoms too often are admitted to
   medical services and exposed to a variety of diagnostic tests
   that yield no improvement in their problems. For the majority

of these patients the root of their problems is psychological, and psychiatric evaluation should precede and usually obviate extensive use of diagnostic tests.[12]

4. The type of payment system does seem to affect utilization of services, and significant differences between fee-for-service and HMO settings in hospital utilization trends have been well documented.[13]

5. There may be too many physicians with surgical privileges in the United States, including approximately 12 percent of the practitioners who are foreign medical graduates.[14] Several studies suggest that unnecessary surgery abounds,[15,16,17,18,19] perhaps as a result of this excessive number of surgeons.

6. Other studies have detected unnecessary long-term care,[20,21] unnecessary admissions,[19,20,21,22,23] unnecessary testing,[24,25,26] and inappropriate antibiotics.[27,28]

To exemplify the problems facing peer evaluation let us examine the issues raised by unnecessary testing. Griner found that during an average fourteen-day stay in the hospital, the patient received sixty-nine laboratory tests, the cost of which comprised 25 percent of the hospital bill. There appeared to be little association between laboratory use and the outcome of care.[29] The potential for waste and abuse in laboratory testing is substantial,[30] much of this being due to misinterpretation of results, technical errors, physiological variations within an individual patient, uncritical acceptance of published opinions, and most flagrant of all, unnecessary repetition of tests.[31] Quality control of laboratory testing done in physicians' offices is an additional problem.[32] One innovative approach to improving laboratory work was undertaken in Canada where 0.5 percent of the fees paid for lab services was withheld to conduct quality assurance within the laboratories themselves.[33]

While financial gain and fear of malpractice are often pointed to as the major factors that underlie high rates of laboratory testing, there are other explanations. McDonald, for example, has shown that clinical errors and subsequent overutilization of lab testing is due not to greed but to the physicians' inability to process the bulk of information presented to them in testing a single case.[34] So far as diagnostic tests are concerned, physicians may be suffering from information overload.

Finally, it was found in an extensive review of medical records that adherence to standards for optimal laboratory testing set by physician members of a PSRO would have produced a 97.8-percent increase in the number of laboratory tests ordered. The study raises serious questions regarding the value of normative criteria in peer review.[35]

Other issues confront peer evaluation experts as well. The choice of location of treatment for a given patient, a factor that affects not only quality of care but also its costs is one of these. Davenport has shown that certain kinds of surgery can be performed as safely and effectively on an ambulatory basis as in the hospital. Similarly, home dialysis is as effective in prolonging life expectancy as institutionally performed dialysis, and it is much less expensive.[36] It is estimated that more than $240 million would be saved yearly if all patients undergoing dialysis had it done at home.

Another is the issue of abuses of third-party reimbursement systems. Peer evaluation must develop strategies for dealing with fraud in billing practices, promiscuous referrals, overutilization of physician services in nursing homes, and so on.[37] Hospital utilization review programs that concentrate too heavily on one segment of the patient population (for example, Medicare patients) to the exclusion of other segments create additional problems as do programs in which there is little coordination between the utilization review committee and other hospital committees working on quality assurance and cost containment.[38]

Will certification and relicensure of physicians improve quality of care and help to reduce costs? Perhaps. In one study it was found that noncertified MDs gave four times as many inappropriate injections as did certified MDs.[39] Likewise, the fact that patient demand and extramedical factors can contribute to unnecessary use of hospitals and other medical services must be recognized. Inability to follow directions, and home situations in which social isolation is a critical problem may contribute significantly to decisions to admit patients to hospitals.[40]

Peer evaluation must also concern itself with the relationship between cost of inpatient care and quality of care. Modern hospitals fully equipped with up-to-date operating rooms, intensive care units, and sophisticated laboratories have become the sina qua non of high-quality care.

It may be that the current approach to quality assurance, concentrating as it does on input of services and the application of modern technology, may have outlived its usefulness to the problem of rising costs and may dictate a more judicious use of health resources.[41]

Ambulatory care in many ways is less well understood than hospital care and well may have a high potential for cost containment. Kessner signaled a major difficulty facing peer evaluation in the ambulatory care sector when he found a twenty-ninefold variation among six ambulatory practice sites in the prevalence of anxiety and depression. He also found serious deficiencies in using encounter forms as compared to medical record abstracts in recording diagnoses. In short, a major challenge facing peer evaluation is to determine what is being done, why, and with what effects.[42] This will be a particular problem for mental health.

Another concern is whether peer evaluation should focus only on utilization of service or whether it should explicitly confront the issue of the prices of the services as well. Rivlin found that price contributed 60 percent of the increase in personal health expenditures between 1950 and 1976,[43] and Rosenthal suggests that changing treatment practices will not have the effect of reducing health care costs. Expenditures for new services and equipment may outweigh the savings from practice reductions.[44] It is worth noting that nearly all Western countries that use fee schedules for reimbursing physician services have eventually adopted schedules that control physician fees through specifying the maximum allowable charge to the patient for a given service.[45] The emphasis in peer evaluation programs thus far has been on the problem of rising utilization. If price is a major contributor to the problem of health care costs, it seems likely that existing peer evaluation efforts will not save much money. An HEW study of PSRO has recently concluded just that. In fact PSROs are expected to cost more than twice as much as Medicare utilization review efforts and achieve no better results as far as cost containment is concerned. In 1978 and beyond pressure on PSROs to show some economic payoffs will almost certainly increase.[46]

This raises a crucial question about peer evaluation in general. Some argue that the cost of conducting quality assurance and peer evaluation programs outweigh benefits except where gross deficiencies in quality or overutilization exist. Quality assurance programs can lead to increased costs in at least three ways: (1) by altering economic incentives, (2) by the increasing utilization as a result of conformance to quality assurance criteria and standards, and (3) by espousing incorrect clinical decision rules that are inflationary without offsetting increases in health benefits.[47] Payne and colleagues, for example, have shown that if quality assurance programs in Hawaii had been successful in increasing physician performance levels to normative standards that had been set, the number of ambulatory services would have increased over 140 percent.[48] Others have found similar results.[49] Thus PSROs by their structures and functions have limited cost control potential and may even help to raise costs. Certainly, any potential of PSROs in cost containment will not be realized unless they are linked with other efforts such as hospital rate review, control of supply, and control of benefit packages.[50]

Clearly there are a number of problems and issues that must be faced by peer evaluation in improving its own techniques as well as in improving quality of care and containing costs.

WHAT CAN PEER EVALUATION DO TO REDUCE COSTS?

The greatest support is given to conducting a profile analysis on each physician. A suggested approach is to start by analyzing several hundred cases of the five most frequent diagnoses in one hospital. Data to be captured for each physician treating patients with these diagnoses would include: physician specialty; care rendered prior to and after hospitalization; length of stay; the frequency of diagnostic testing; and patient outcomes as indicated by discharge status. Any study of this type should also control for patient mix. The purpose would be to identify variations in practice and to use the results as an educational tool.

Results would be presented to individual physicians with the understanding that some confidentiality is desirable and with the expectation that almost invariably there will be defensive reactions by some physicians. Physicians who are outliers in the sense of using above average numbers of tests or other services would receive special attention in efforts to change their behavior through feedback and other behavior modification techniques. The essence of the approach is to compile objective data on practice patterns and apply peer pressure to those physicians whose practice patterns lie outside the norms. The chief of service should have the detailed breakdowns on utilization and use these in discussions with physicians.

It is acknowledged that empirical norms do not necessarily indicate good quality. Concurrent efforts, therefore, would be made to evaluate existing practices so as to develop criteria that would reflect the most cost-effective clinical decision making. Ultimately enforcement of these criteria could be linked to the payment system.

Two other efforts, which are regarded as crucial to peer evaluation's role in cost containment, are to more adequately define what a peer is and to expand upon the concept of the second opinion. Many physicians are convinced that peer evaluation committees, in order to be maximally effective, should be heterogeneous. That is, various specialties should review the same case because they can bring in different perspectives. Homogeneous committees (for example, all internists on the same committee) may inordinately reflect the bias of their own specialty. In summary, there should be a broader basis for determining who a peer is when the task is to develop criteria and improve quality.

The next greatest cost containment potential was felt to lie with second opinions required of all specialties admitting patients to the hospital. There is additional support for the notion of having a pre-admission or postdischarge second opinion, or both, to confirm the need for the length of stay. The second-opinion program could eventually be linked to the payment structure. Clearly, the strongest motivation in peer pressure is that of payment denial.

A number of other potential areas of pursuit for peer evaluation include the following:

Audit by diagnosis or cost rather than conducting reviews of a given practice.

Commence peer evaluation training at the residency level.

Conduct extensive evaluations of ancillary testing to determine why tests are reported during admission; what effects extensive diagnostic workups have on the elderly or dying patients; degrees of superfluous data presented to physicians by serial testing and standing orders; reasons for variations between hospitals in admission screening tests; the physician's capacity to deal with diagnostic test data and ways to improve that capacity.

Increase physician accountability for overutilization at the hospital level. First, the physician could be made financially responsible for unnecessary treatments. Second, selected services could be capitated to discourage unnecessary utilization.

Improve professional competence in terms of cognitive knowledge as well as demonstrating skills and judgment through improved competency and skills exams.

Direct studies of the negative effects of treatment on a patient's health. Most often, the effects of overutilization of services on patients are not addressed even though they may have important implications for quality assurance.

Establish guidelines for appropriate referrals. Much ambulatory laboratory and x-ray work is done on a self-referred basis. The potential for conflict of interest is high and bears investigation and, possibly, control. Both the danger of unnecessary repeated testing and of inadequate quality control measures should be recognized.

Establish primary care referral guidelines. Many patients being treated by primary care physicians have psychological, not medical, problems, and patients with psychiatric diagnoses are known to be high utilizers of medical services.[51] Psychiatric intervention has been shown to reduce subsequent medical care utilization and save money.[52] Early referral to mental health professionals may improve patient outcomes and also save money.

Establish a quality assurance data base for use in cost-effective clinical decision making. The SOSSUS study of the American College of Surgeons, for example, suggested the establishment of an ongoing system to collect, analyze, and report data on morbidity and the economic cost of illness that could help shape expenditures for health.

Measure changes in physicians' practice patterns before and after they have been exposed to some form of peer evaluation. Peer review must determine which incentives and methods are the most effective in changing behavior.

Review the costs of conducting peer evaluation activities. Some approaches to peer evaluation are much more costly than others and not necessarily more effective.

Consider both utilization and price increases in peer evaluation, given the latter plays a significant role in health care cost increases.

Encourage studies on the relationship between cost and quality. Increased costs do not necessarily increase quality.

Assist in starting cost containment committees in hospitals and peer review organizations.

Determine medical necessity for each treatment. Given the explosion in medical technology there should be a peer committee looking at old or outmoded procedures and those that are done in combination with other procedures that are redundant or produce no new information.

Conduct more review of ambulatory care.

Encourage third-party endorsement for national peer review in the private sector.

Develop counter strategies for fraud and abuse.

The medical sector needs to have moral and ethical guidelines enunciated by society in reference to the provision of medical care. Death is the last clinical diagnosis; and even death seems difficult to define these days. If that is so, definition of "life" and appropriate attempts to preserve it create even more difficult problems. Somewhere, sometime, the role of medical care in the happiness and productivity of people must be more critically considered by our citizens, not as a medical question, but in a social, moral, and ethical context. Most of us do not want to find ourselves in the position of England in which medical care is rationed across-the-board by laypersons who deny modern medical care to those who, if they had it, could become happier and more productive. We, nevertheless, must face up to the inescapable fact that when there is an insatiable demand for services and a finite limit on resources, there must be some form of rationing.

Peer evaluation can contribute to what one might call "rational rationing," but it is important to emphasize that its use to ration the delivery of medical care must be preceded by clear directives from society as to when and how and under what circumstances it wishes medical care to be provided to the citizens of the United States.

Dr. David Owen provides peer evaluation with its major charge:

> Clinical freedom is not an abstract concept. Its full realization demands that the profession faces the practical economic facts of life. The constraint on the total resources available means that doctors acting individually can constrain the clinical freedom of their colleagues and also limit the effectiveness of health care for other patients. We need a readiness amongst individual doctors to insure that their own particular group of patients does not use up a disproportionate share of available resources at the expense of services to other groups of patients and therefore of the clinical freedom of other doctors. This will not be achieved unless we abandon the self-defeating limited interpretation of clinical freedom as freedom to prescribe treatment for individual patients without regard to the consequences for other patients. . . . Clinical freedom likewise means responsibility, the responsibility of involvement and the responsibility of choosing priorities in health care.[24]

REFERENCES

1. Isele, W. P. Legal aspects of peer review. *The Advocate*, September 1977.
2. Codman, E. A. *The Shoulder* (Rupture of the supraspinatus tendon and other lesions in or about the subacromial bursa). Boston, 1932.
3. *American Medical Association: Peer Review Manual.* Chicago, American Medical Association, May 1971.
4. Williamson, John W. Formulating priorities for quality assurance activity—description of a method and its application, *J.A.M.A.*, 239, 7:631–637, Feb. 12, 1978.
5. Brown, C. B. Assessing quality of patient care—the bi-cycle concept. In E. Scheye (ed), Proceedings of the fifteenth annual symposium on hospital affairs, University of Chicago, May 1973.
6. Brook, R. H. *Quality of Care Assessment—A Comparison of Five Methods of Peer Review.* DHEW, July 1973.

7. Brook. R. H. A study of methodological problems associated with assessment of quality of care. Johns Hopkins University, May 1972.

8. Blankenhorn, M. A. Standards of practice of internal medicine and methods of assessing the quality of practice in hospitals. Editorial, *Ann. Intern. Med.*, 47:367–374, August 1957.

9. Browning, F. E. The record in hospital bed utilization. In *American Medical Association: Utilization Review: A Handbook for the Medical Staff.* American Medical Association, 1965, pp. 77–82.

10. Mitchell, William E. How to deal with poor medical care. *J.A.M.A.*, 236: 2875–2877, Dec. 20, 1976.

11. Aydelotte, M. K., and Tener, M. E. An investigation of the relation between nursing activity and patient welfare. Ames, State University of Iowa, 440, 1960.

12. Goshen, C. E. Diagnostic overkill and management of psychiatric problems. *Men. Hyg.*, 54:306–309, April 1970.

13. Eisenberg, J. M., Whitney, A. M., Kahn, L. T., et al. Patterns of pediatric practice by the same physicians in a prepaid and fee-for-service setting. *Clin. Res.*, 20, 4:736, 1972.

14. *The Study on Surgical Services for the United States (SOSSUS).* Sponsored by American College of Surgeons and the American Surgical Association. Washington, D.C., U.S. Government Printing Office, 1975.

15. Bunker, J. P. Surgical manpower—A comparison of operations and surgeons in the United States and in England and Wales. *N. Engl. J. Med.*, 282, 3: 135–144, Jan. 15, 1970.

16. Doyle, J. C. Unnecessary hysterectomies: Study of 6,248 operations in 35 hospitals during 1948. *J.A.M.A.*, 151:360–365, Jan. 31, 1953.

17. Bolande, R. P. Ritualistic surgery: Circumcision and tonsillectomy. *N. Engl. J. Med.*, 280, 11:591–596, Mar. 13, 1969.

18. Harding, H. E. A notable source of error in the diagnosis of appendicitis. *Brit. Med. J.*, 2: 1028–1029, Oct. 20, 1962.

19. McCarthy, E. G., and Kamons, A. S. Voluntary and mandatory presurgical screening programs: An analysis of their implications. *Clin. Res.*, April 1975.

20. Cristo, C. Surveyor opinion, development and implementation in Monroe County, New York. *J.A.M.A.*, 196, 12:1065–1066, June 20, 1966.

21. Duff, R. S., Cook, C. D., and Wanerka, G. R. Use of utilization review to assess the quality of pediatric inpatient care. *Pediatrics*, 49:169–176, Feb., 1972.

22. Koremic, J., and Perlman, L. V. Preventability of hospital admissions. *Clin. Res.*, 19, 3:662, 1971.

23. Lovejoy, F. H. Unnecessary and preventable hospitalization: Report of an internal audit. *Pediatrics*, 79, 5:868–878, Nov. 1971.

24. Owens, David. Clinical freedom and professional freedom. *Lancet*, 1:1006–1009, May 8, 1976.

25. Paulus, H. E., Coutts, A., and Calabro, J. J. Clinical significance of hyperuricemia in routinely screened hospitalized men. *J.A.M.A.* 211:277–281, Jan. 12, 1970.

26. Bell, R. S., and Loop, J. W. The utility and futility of radiographic skull examination for trauma. *N. Engl. J. Med.*, 284, 5:236–239, Feb. 4, 1971.
27. Barker, K. N., Kimbrough, W. W., and Heller, W. M. A study of medication errors in a hospital. University of Mississippi, Mar. 1968.
28. Brucker, P., Brown, C, and Gonnella, J. Diagnosis before therapy: A model in physicians continuing education. *J. Med. Educ.*, 44, 10:980–981, Oct. 1969.
29. Griner, Paul F., and Liptzin, Benjamin. Use of the laboratory in a teaching hospital. *Ann. Intern. Med.*, 75: 157–163, 1971.
30. Fineberg, Harvey. Clinical chemistries: The high cost of low-cost diagnostic tests. In S. Altman and R. Blendon (eds.), *Medical Technologies: The Culprit Behind Health Care Costs?* DHEW, Sept. 1979.
31. Zieve, Leslie. Misinterpretation and abuse of laboratory tests by clinicians. *Ann. N.Y. Acad. Sci.*, 134:564–572, 1966.
32. Schoen, I., Thomas, G. D., and Lance, S. The quality of performance in physicians' office laboratories. *Am. J. Clin. Pathol.*, 55:163–170, Feb. 1971.
33. Bell, R. E. Medical laboratory accreditation and quality control in Alberta: I. Laboratory accreditation. *Can. Med. Assoc. J.*, 103, 11:L1169–1174, 1970.
34. McDonald, Clement. Protocol-based computer reminders, the quality of care and the nonperfectability of man. *N. Engl. J. Med.*, 294, 24:1351–1355, Dec. 9, 1976.
35. Gordon, D. L., Howell, E., and Fuller, M. A. PSRO effect on frequency of laboratory testing. Washington, D.C., National Capital Medical Foundation, April 1976.
36. Stange, Paul V., and Andrew, T. Summer. Predicting treatment costs and life expectancy for end-stage renal disease. *N. Engl. J. Med.*, 298:372–378, Feb. 16, 1978.
37. Bellin, L. E., and Cavaler, F. Medicaid practitioner and abuses and excuses vs. counterstrategy of New York City health department. *Am. J. of Pub. Health*, 61, 11:2201–2210, Nov. 1971.
38. Berman, L. T., Dvorschock, K. T., and Smith, D. D. Utilization review in Connecticut hospitals: Three years after Medicare. Yale University, 1969.
39. Brook, R. H., and Williams, K. N. Evaluation of the New Mexico peer review system, 1971 to 1973. *Med. Care*, 14 (12 Suppl.), Dec. 1976.
40. Mushlin, A. I., and Appel, F. A. Extramedical factors in the decision to hospitalize medical patients. *Am. J. Pub. Health*, 66, 2:170–172, Feb. 1976.
41. Gellman, D. D. Cost-benefit in health care: We need to know much more. *Cal. Med. Assoc. J.*, 3:988–989, Nov. 2, 1974.
42. Kessner, D. M. Quality assessment and assurance: Early signs of cognitive dissonance. *N. Engl. J. Med.*, 298, 7:381–386, Feb. 16, 1978.
43. Rivlin, Alice M. Expenditures for health care: Federal programs and their effects. Congress of the United States, Government Printing Office, Aug. 1977.
44. Rosenthal, Gerald. Controlling the cost of health care. National Center for Health Services Research policy research series, Rockville, Md., May 1977.

45. Anderson, Odin W. All health care systems struggle against rising costs. *Hospitals*, 50:92–102, Oct. 1, 1976.
46. Peck, R. L. Will this be the year they kill PSROs? *Med. Econ.*, p. 35, Jan. 23, 1978.
47. Phelps, C. Benefit—cost analysis of quality assurance programs. In Richard H. Egdahl and Paul Gertman (eds.), *Quality Assurance in Health Care.* Germantown, Md., Aspen Systems Corp., 1976.
48. Payne, B. E., and Study Staff, Lyons, T. F., et al. The quality of medical care: Evaluation and improvement. *Hospital Research and Educational Trust.* Chicago, 1976.
49. Brook, Robert H., and Davies-Avery, Allyson. Quality assurance and cost control. In G. A. Giebink and N. H. White (eds.), *Ambulatory Medical Care Quality Assurance 1977, Issues, Directions and Applications.* La Jolla, Calif.: La Jolla Health Science Publications, 1977.
50. Egdahl, R. H., Gertman, Paul, Taft, Cynthia, and Giller, Ronald. Quality assurance in hospitals: Policy alternatives. Report of a conference on quality assurance in hospitals, Boston, November 21-22, 1975. Boston, Springer International Publications, April 1976.
51. Anderson, R., Francis, Anita, Lion, Joanna, and Doughety, Virginia. Psychologically related illness and health service utilization, *Med. Care*, 15:5, 59–73, May 1977.
52. Karon, B. P., and Vanden Bos, Gary R. Treatment costs of psychotherapy versus medication for schizophrenics. *Prof. Psychol.*, 293–298, Aug. 1975.

PART IV

Clinical Decisions

Chapter 8

Cost-effective Clinical Decision Making

Duncan Neuhauser*
William B. Stason†

Traditional clinical decision making does not explicitly assume resource scarcity. The goal of the physician is to do everything that can be done for each patient following the slogan that "nothing is too good for my patient."

Cost-effective clinical decision making (CECDM) explicitly assumes scarcity. It is understood that resources used for this patient are not available for that patient. The goal is to maximize the benefits of medical care for a defined population given a limited amount of resources, such as doctors' time, hospital beds, blood, and drugs. It means doing less than the maximum for some patients in order to save resources for the greater benefit of several other patients.

Cost-effective clinical decision making (CECDM) may sound like a very new idea, but in fact physicians practice it all the time. Here is an explanation of how it happens.

The first patient a medical student works up may take that student six hours. The history and physical are slow, methodical, and

*Associate Professor of Health Services Administration, Harvard School of Public Health.

†Associate Professor of Health Services Administration, Center for the Analysis of Health Practices, Harvard School of Public Health; Veteran's Administration Outpatient Clinic, Boston.

exhaustive. That student soon goes on to a clinical rotation and is asked to work up six patients in six hours. The student does not learn to speak six times faster; he or she reduces the number of questions to those assumed to have a high probability of finding a significant correctable problem. If the student finds a significant problem with one of these patients, he or she may well spend more time with that patient and less time with other patients. The student has discovered resource scarcity: namely, time, and thus attempting to allocate this scarce resource so as to get the most benefit to the population of six patients. Time spent with the first patient is not available to spend with patients two through six. This student has learned to practice cost-effective clinical decision making by force of circumstance. Are the patients upset? No. It probably takes an unusual, carefully selected patient who will tolerate a six-hour history and physical. Patients understand that a doctor has many people to take care of, and nearly all patients accept this fact.

So why discuss cost-effective clinical decision making? As we hope to show, not every physician practices CECDM as well as he or she might. It is learned by force of circumstances. What is kept and what is dropped depends on the physician and the custom that prevails in the clinical setting in which this physician works.

For each question and each test there might be tables of probabilities that vary by patient age, sex, and clinical setting. There might be estimates of the costs of pursuing such medical interventions to compare with the benefits. It might be a systematic approach but most likely it is not.

Should a blood pressure be taken? If it is evaluated, what further testing is called for? What are the benefits from treatment, less the side effects? What is the likelihood the patient will comply with a medical regimen? Is it better for this patient simply to lose weight, reduce the intake of salt, and sign up for transcendental meditation, or should medicine be prescribed?

Some of these essential items of information will be known by the student whereas others will not, and some will simply be guessed at. We would contend that there are analytic techniques that can help make this approach to CECDM systematic. These techniques derive from epidemiology, statistics, economics management, operations research, and an applied branch of mathematics called decision analysis.

1. A favorite example of cost-ineffective clinical decision making is that of Dr. Harvey Cushing at Ypres. Dr. Cushing was a noted Harvard neurosurgeon who went to Yale in the first part of this century, and Ypres was a battlefield in World War I. Cushing was an army surgeon in the war. Although the allied mortality was as much

as 50,000 on some days, not counting the wounded, Cushing operated very carefully on only two patients a day.

2. A second example of cost-ineffective clinical decision making, however, is something we can change. They are the weekly case records published in the *New England Journal of Medicine*, which were founded by Richard C. Cabot.

A very large battery of laboratory tests are carried out and presented. The expert physician has two weeks to study these findings. It is rumored to be bad form for the expert to complain that too few tests were ordered. The expert summarizes the key findings and draws a set of conclusions. Then the truth is expounded by a pathologist who gives the correct answer (*New Engl. J. Med.*, 297:8, 455). Everyone realizes that this is a highly stylized, ritualized performance that gives fame to everyone involved. Are all the (often invasive) tests necessary? According to Dr. Marvin Shapiro, in referring to the June 23, 1977, case:

> The tomograms fluoroscopy and studies of the barium filled esophagus, in my opinion, contributed nothing of importance to the care of the patient. I certainly find no value in the computed tomographic scan. True, the CT scan demonstrated that the probably benign anterior mediastinal lesion contained a large amount of fat. This bit of information stimulated a certain amount of intellectual activity but in no way affected the clinical course. Including the extra days in the hospital which were required to accomplish the radiological studies, an estimate of an unnecessary $1,000 of cost seems conservative.

There might be additional probability estimates. To quote Dr. W. K. Morgan, another recent critic of these cases:

> How often does one see lymphangitic carcinomatosis in the absence of pulmonary symptoms or signs.

It is understood that these cases often have unusual outcomes. A test is negative when usually it would be positive. How often does this happen?

> Surely the essence of good medical practice is expeditious diagnosis and treatment with the patient undergoing a minimum of discomfort. Do we not have an obligation to keep the patient's hospital bill to a minimum?

Should the reward not go to making the diagnosis as efficiently and painlessly as possible, rather than to "erudite discussions" of low probability and unusual events. Each of these reports should indicate what the patient's bill was. Each of these reports should estimate the magnitude of the benefits that resulted from treatment. Benefits to treatment should be the payoff and diagnosis an intermediate way station, not an end in itself.

Instead of attempting to explain the assumptions and logic behind CECDM, it is easier to give some examples. Let us begin by looking for colon cancer; after that we will turn to hypertension.

Before discussing colon cancer, let us make clear the difference between clinical decisions and research findings. When one comes from the perspective of decision analysis, one is struck with physicians' commitment to numerical facts and lack of explicit concern for the process by which clinical decisions are arrived at. The nature of clinical decisions is that they have to be made in the absence of perfect knowledge. This is in contrast to research. A researcher can spend an entire lifetime on one problem and never find an answer. Since perfect information rarely exists, clinical decisions must be made based in part on research evidence and in part on "guesstimates." Physicians seem uncomfortable about the guesstimates that they have to make all the time.

In the colon cancer example that follows, the numbers are very approximate. They are rounded off and simplified so as to make the process of analysis comprehensible. Any gastroenterologist might bring his or her expert judgment to bear and substitute the "right" numbers.

The hypertension example that follows is one in which a lot of effort has gone into finding the "best" numbers and working through the analysis. The colon cancer example is "quick and dirty" or clinical. The hypertension example is extensive, academic, and could be labeled as "research." Few practicing physicians would do such detailed research analysis although they may be consumers of such information. In short, there is a method in the numerical madness that follows.

COST-EFFECTIVE DECISION
MAKING IN COLON CANCER

First, does early detection in asymptomatic colon cancer make a difference? What evidence do we have that the patient might benefit from it? There is one randomized trial relevant to this question for which we are indebted to Dr. Morris Collin and the Epidemiology Research Unit of Kaiser Permanente in Oakland. The study is not well known because it was published in the *Information in Medicine Journal* from Stuttgart, Germany. This study undertook to see if yearly multiphasic screening would make a difference in mortality. Four thousand patients were randomized into two groups. One group of patients was encouraged to undergo screening. The other group was not encouraged. A seven-year followup showed that for only two diseases was mortality significantly reduced: colon cancer and hypertension. One can conclude from this that multiphasic screening is not cost effective, but looking for colon cancer and hypertension is effective. But is it cost effective? Is it worth the effort?

Consider the different possible primary tests for detecting asymptomatic colon cancer:

Occult blood (OB)
Sigmoidoscopy (SIG)
Digital examination (DE)
Colonoscopy (COL)

In the analysis that follows, other tests such as barium enema are not considered. They are assumed to be followup tests to be used after a positive primary test. The reader may wish to change these assumptions and redo the analysis.

Occult blood testing is an inexpensive and noninvasive test. Other tests are increasingly more costly and have increased risks. Table 8.1 summarizes the costs and effectiveness of these tests in detecting

Table 8.1. Tests to Detect Colon Cancer (CA), Their Estimated Costs, and Percent of Cancers Found

OB	
$1	Finds 75% of all colonic CAs
DE	
$2	Finds 90% of the 10% of colonic CAs that occur in the rectum
SIG	
$20	Finds all of the 60% of colonic CAs that occur in the rectosigmoid
(There is some small risk with the use of sigmoidoscopy)	
COL	
$250	Finds all CAs that are findable.
(This procedure has risks)	

colon cancer whereas Figure 8.1 represents the same information in diagrammatic form. The entire rectangle represents 100 percent of detectable rectal and colon cancers. OB is assumed to find 75 percent of these cancers throughout the whole range of the lower intestinal tract. This assumes that some cancers never bleed at all and will be undetectable by occult blood. This figure of 75 percent is a sheer guess. Information about this critical number is not known but is essential to answering the problem. It turns out that the analysis is very "sensitive" to differences in this number. This is a good example of how clinical decisions must proceed in the absence of good research data. Although DE is assumed to find 90 percent of cancers in the lower end (rectum), only 10 percent of all cancers are found in this area. Thus, the digital exam will fine only nine cancers out of 100. However, SIG is assumed to find all cancers within its range, and COL is presumed to find 100 percent of detectable cancers.

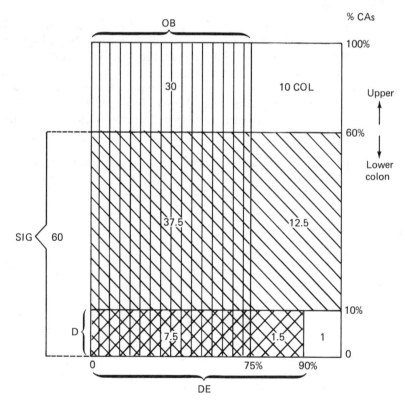

Figure 8-1. Diagram of range of tests for colon cancer (CA).

There well may be cancers that are undetectable by any test, but since they cannot be found, they can be ignored in our analysis.

It is not sufficient to know that early detection of colon cancer prolongs life. How much is life prolonged per patient with asymptomatic cancer thus detected? An analysis of the National Cancer Institute survival curves suggests that life is prolonged on the average about four years per patient.

One way to structure this problem is to consider a rank order of these tests from lowest cost, lowest yield to highest cost, highest yield. OB costs the least and COL the most. Because DE and SIG are higher cost and lower yield than OB, they can be rejected from consideration. If you could do only one of these tests, OB would be preferred.

However, consider the following combinations:

OB&DE
OB&SIG

These fall in between OB and COL. Table 8.2 shows these four options in order from lowest yield (75) to highest yield (100).

Let us assume that in this particular population there is one cancer to be found per 100 patients or 100 cancers per 10,000 patients. Further consider the problem of false positives (the test says cancer but further testing shows no cancer). Assume OB has 500 false positives; OB&DE 550 positives; OB&SIG 500 false positives; and COL no false positives. What is the cost of further testing required to separate true positives from false positives? Assume these costs are $400 for OB and OB&D and $380 for OB&S.

We are now in a position to calculate the total costs for each of these four strategies (see Table 8.3). The numbers in Table 8.3 can be

Table 8.2. Four Possible Primary Tests for Asymptomatic Colon Cancer; Their True Positives, False Positives, and Costs

	True Positives	False Positives	$ Per Patient (primary test only)
OB	75	500	1
OB&DE	76.5	550	3
OB&SIG	90	500	21
COL	100	0	250

Note: These numbers are for a population of 10,000 people and assume one cancer per 100 people.

Table 8.3. Total Costs per 10,000 Patients for Four Strategies for Detection of Colon Cancer

Strategy	Costs of Basic Test	Costs of Removing False Positives	Total Costs
OB	10,000 X $1 = $10,000	(500 + 75)($400) = $230,000	$240,000
OB&DE	10,000 X $3 = $30,000	(550 + 76.5)($400) = $250,600	$280,600
OB&SIG	10,000 X $21 = $210,000	(500 + 90)($380) = $224,200	$434,200
COL	10,000 X $250 = $2,500,000	0	$2,500,000

divided by 10,000 to obtain the cost per patient. If the reader finds this more appealing, the resultant analysis will not change.

Now we can consider the marginal cost per cancer found. The marginal cost is the additional cost to find an additional case as one moves along the scale of increased costs. This is shown in Table 8.4. The first seventy-five cancers can be found by OB at a cost of $3200 per cancer found. The next one and a half cancers can be found by moving to OB&D at a marginal cost of $27,066 per cancer found. The next 13.5 cancers can be found at $11,377. Since $11,377 is greater than $27,066, the OB&DE can be excluded from consideration. If one were willing to spend $27,066 the next 13.5 cancers could be found. Thus we can eliminate OB&DE from consideration. This is done in Table 8.5. Going from OB to OB&SIG finds fifteen more cancers at a marginal cost of $12,946 per additional cancer found. Going from OB&SIG to COL as the first test for all patients costs $206,580 per cancer found at the margin. Since we assumed that each case of cancer found will prolong life by four years on the average, we can divide the marginal costs per cancer found in the upper part of Table 8.5 to obtain the marginal cost per year of life saved.

Table 8.4. Marginal Cost per Cancer Found, Four Strategies

Strategy	Additional Numbers of Cancers Found	Additional Costs	Marginal Cost per Cancers Found
OB	75	$240,000	$3200
OB&DE	1.5	40,600	27,066
OB&SIG	13.5	153,600	11,377
COL	10	2,065,800	206,580

Table 8.5. Marginal Cost per Cancer Found and per Year of Life Saved

	Additional Cancers Found	Additional Costs	Marginal Cost Per CA Found	Marginal Cost per Year of Life Saved
OB	75	240,000	$3200	$800
OB&SIG	15	194,200	12,946	3236
COL	10	2,065,800	206,580	51,645

Note: Based on a population of 10,000 patients with one cancer per 100 patients and four years of life saved per cancer found.

How much is too much to spend per year of life saved? One could pick a number, for example, $15,000 per year of life saved, as a cutoff point. If so, OB&SIG would be justified, assuming our numbers are correct, but COL for all 10,000 people would not be.

A second way to approach this problem would be to assume that a single practicing physician can practice medicine on the average of fifty hours per week. The time will be allocated to activities with the highest benefit to cost ratio, and the "last" activity to be undertaken before the fifty hours is used up becomes the marginal cost per year of life saved, which becomes the cutoff point. Assume that the last hours could be filled up doing OB&SIG; $3236 would then be the cutoff point. If an activity with a higher cost per year of life saved came along, it would not be done. If lower, it would be done. Thus, it is quite possible that a suburban doctor may have a different cutoff point from a doctor in a rural area in which there are many more patients per doctor.

SENSITIVITY ANALYSIS

We would be greatly disappointed if the reader remembered only the numerical result rather than the method and approach. It is our hope that the reader would replace our numbers with those more to his or her liking and recalculate. See what happens to marginal costs if OB detected 90 percent rather than 75 percent of cancers found. See what happens if there is one cancer per 1000 rather than one per hundred. Slightly more complicated problems are as follows: What about the side effects associated with colonoscopy? This could affect both cost and benefit sides of the ratio. The side effects result in added costs of treatment that should be added to the cost side. The side effects such as a perforated intestine should be subtracted from the "benefit" side. Assume that in a population of 10,000 there would be one perforation per 1000 patients. Would it be better to avoid a perforation or to find a cancer? Assume that finding a cancer is worth the risk of two perforations. The ten perforations can then be turned into five cancer equivalents, and the marginal benefits of COL are reduced from ten, less these five cancer equivalents, to five. By halving the marginal cases found, the marginal costs per case double to over $400,000.

What about doing these screening tests yearly? Prevalent cancers found on the first screen are removed from the population, and only incident cases occurring during the year are available for detection next year. What about detection and removal of polyps? This requires equating polyps with cancers. This might be calculated on the basis of the probability that a polyp becomes a cancer. Because this would happen in the future, their removal would result in a future benefit that may not be as highly valued as a benefit obtained today. The jargon term for adjusting for costs and benefits occurring at different times is called "discounting to present value" or just "discounting."

We can now define a physician who practices cost-effective clinical decision making as one who, given a choice, will take on the activity with the lowest cost per quality-adjusted year of life saved.

Now let us consider the following examples of physician behavior related to seeking colon cancer that do not fit this definition of cost-effective clinical decision making:

1. The American Cancer Society recommends OB, DE, and either SIG or COL yearly for all adults over the age of forty. They propose a marginal cost per year of life saved that may be somewhere between $3000 and $500,000 per year of life saved.
2. One group of physicians in an HMO familiar with the Morris Collin study were doing SIG yearly without OB. Although they were convinced that life could be prolonged, they were faced with a financial crunch and abandoned SIG altogether. They decided it was not "worth it." They did not replace SIG with OB. They did nothing except for patients admitted to the hospital. These patients were tested for OB routinely. These tests have high false positives that can be reduced by controlling diet (e.g., not eating rare or raw meat). Because so many procedures were being administered to these inpatients, they could not control their diet. Any patient with a positive test result was sent for a barium enema. An alternative would have been to guaiac test prior to admission; if the result were positive,

the test should be repeated under dietary control; if it is still positive, SIG or COL, or both, should be ordered. Instead of reducing expensive false positives in this way, these inpatients were given barium enema exams, which may well have extended their hospital stay for one day.

3. When teaching a group of Scandinavian physician managers some time ago, the question of looking for colon cancer was raised. All the physicians agreed that the yield was too small to be worth the effort. They were amazed to discover that they were not thereby willing to spend $800 per year of life saved. They had not bothered with such simple calculations.

4. A noted eastern teaching hospital used benzadine tests to seek occult blood rather than stool guaiac. If the test were positive a barium enema was ordered. The benzadine test had a very high rate of false positives. For every true positive there were fifty false positives. This was part of the cause of a major bottleneck in radiology. Outpatient barium enemas had a two-week waiting time. Radiology was fully aware of the problem, but felt they were helpless in changing the behavior of hospital physicians.

5. Another HMO primary care group decided on one stool guaiac test yearly combined with DE for women only, since this test was associated with a routine yearly pelvic exam. A rational strategy perhaps, except that if the stool guaiac were positive, a barium enema was ordered without a repeat guaiac with dietary control.

6. A noted clinic published a report of several thousand SIG on asymptomatic patients. They failed to check how many of the true positives would have been found by OB, which could have been a very simple additional study. Their published paper concluded that yearly SIG was worthwhile. In private conversation one of the authors said they were thinking of abandoning SIG as too much effort for too little yield.

We trust that by now the point is clear. Looking for colon cancer can be cost effective. Although we would be happy to pay $800 per year of life saved, in each case the decision rules that were used were not explicitly thought out and were nonoptimal as a result.

We would like to think that physicians could go through the kind of calculations that we have described and develop strategies consistent with their population and economic context. There is no right answer for everyone and every setting. That is why approximate numbers here do not bother us.

We would like physicians to learn how to "push" these numbers and draw their own conclusions, to learn the process of decision making and not simply the answer. New and better numbers will hopefully be reported with this simple analysis recalculated over and over again.

Now let us leave this purposely oversimplified analysis for a discussion of hypertension.

COST-EFFECTIVE DECISION MAKING IN HYPERTENSION

There are two fundamental—and obvious—underpinnings for cost-effective decision making. One is the need for objective assessment of the *effectiveness* of health practices or procedures and the other is awareness of the true *costs* of these practices or procedures—costs in terms of human resources, materials, or dollars. Unfortunately, neither criterion is met with any consistency in current medical practice. All too often physicians have been shown to be unaware of the costs of the laboratory examinations they order, the daily charges for hospital beds or operating rooms, and the costs of medications they prescribe for their patients. *Improved cost awareness is the first prerequisite for cost-effective decision making.*

Second, there are many medical practices, some extremely popular, for which criteria for proper application are not fully established. Amongst these I would number tonsillectomy, breast cancer surgery, coronary bypass surgery, CAT scanners, and coronary care units. It is not that these practices are ineffective; it is only that they are either of unproven effectiveness or that patient characteristics for their selective application have not been well defined. Unfortunately, once such practices become established, the momentum they create becomes very difficult to modify. Even studies to evaluate them become difficult or impossible. *So evaluation of effectiveness is the second cornerstone of cost-effective decision making.* For the practitioner this usually means critical use of available literature in judging the effectiveness of a given procedure for a given patient; for the academician it means generating the required study to establish its effectiveness.

Careful weighing of the balance between costs and effectiveness is cost-effective decision making. Our analysis of hypertension management makes use of these principles.[1]

First, why hypertension? Hypertension is an important health problem. It affects over 24 million people, and treatment, if offered to all, would cost nearly $5 billion per year. Furthermore, treatment, though clearly efficacious for some men, is of uncertain value in two-thirds of the patients with mild hypertension and in women.

Data for our study were drawn widely from the clinical, epidemiological, and health statistics literature. Reliance was placed on the Framingham Heart Study for estimates of the morbidity and mortality resulting from elevated blood pressure (BP).[2,3] Although imperfect, we feel that the data used represent the best available.

To develop a model for hypertension management, we first specified costs, most importantly, the costs of treating hypertension (medications, physician fees, and laboratory tests) and the medical care cost savings from the strokes and myocardial infarctions (MIs) prevented. Then we calculated expected benefits in terms of the improved life expectancy adjusted for estimated effects on the quality of life or morbidity prevented and of the adverse effects of medication side effects. Quality of life adjustments were based on the concept that a year of life with angina or the residuum of a stroke is worth something less to the individual than a year of life or full health. Finally, net costs were related to net benefits to obtain our measure of cost effectiveness in dollars per quality-adjusted year of life saved.

Where data were particularly sparse, the effects of a number of alternative assumptions on the results were tested—in what is called sensitivity analysis. This technique provides a means to identify critical weak lines in the analysis and to target priorities for future research. The most important weak link in our opinion, is our inadequate knowledge of the degree of benefit to be expected from treating hypertension, especially mild hypertension (diastolic BP ≤ 105 mm Hg). To deal with this problem, we made several assumptions about the degree of risk reduction that might be expected from treatment, ranging from no benefit to full benefit. Full benefit implies full reduction of risk of a hypertensive patient to that of a person who has had a normal BP all of his or her life. As can be imagined, results depend importantly on which assumption is chosen.

A few examples will serve to illustrate our results.

Table 8.6 shows estimated gains in life expectancy from treating patients whose diastolic BPs are lowered from 110 to 90 mm Hg. Considerable differences can be seen between a full-benefit assumption (FB) and an age-varying benefit (AVPB). In age-varying partial benefit, treatment is assumed to be more effective if it is begun earlier in life. The effect of this assumption is particularly noticeable in older men and women. We believe the age-varying benefit assumption is probably closer to the truth.

Table 8.6. Increase in Life Expectancy and Quality-adjusted Life Expectancy According to Age and Sex

Age (years)	Life Expectancy (years)	Increase in Life Expectancy (years)		Increase in Quality-Adjusted Life Expectancy (years)	
		FB	Average FB	FB	Average FB
Women					
20	53.2	5.0	4.7	5.4	5.0
30	43.9	4.4	3.8	4.8	4.1
40	34.8	3.7	2.6	4.0	2.8
50	26.4	2.8	1.7	3.1	1.9
60	18.5	2.3	1.0	2.6	1.2
Men					
20	46.5	8.1	6.9	8.2	7.1
30	38.2	5.8	4.1	5.9	4.2
40	29.7	3.9	2.2	4.0	2.3
50	21.7	2.5	1.0	2.6	1.1
60	14.5	1.4	0.3	1.5	0.4

Source: M. Weinstein and W. Stason, Allocation of resources to manage hypertension, New Engl. J. Med., 296:735, March 31, 1977. Reprinted by permission from The New England Journal of Medicine.
Note: FB = fraction of benefit.

In Figure 8.2 the cost effectiveness in dollars per quality-adjusted life year of life is plotted against pretreatment diastolic BP for women and men according to the age at which treatment is begun. The cost effectiveness of treatment varies from less than $4000 to more than $50,000 per year of life saved; is better at higher initial levels of diastolic BP; and, for males, becomes less cost effective with increasing age while, for women, the converse is true. This difference between the sexes can be explained by the fact that the complications of arteriosclerosis occur later in life in women than in men. If a $10,000 cutoff per year of life saved were chosen as a criterion for treatment, one would treat twenty-year-old men whose diastolic BP was about 90 mm Hg and sixty-year-old men only if their diastolic BP reached 118 mm Hg or higher.

Figure 8.2 showed the results of cost effectiveness assuming that patients maintain treatment throughout their lives and take their medications with sufficient regularity to actually achieve BP control. Frequently, however, nonadherence is a significant problem. Under reasonable assumptions about the degree of expected adherence, the

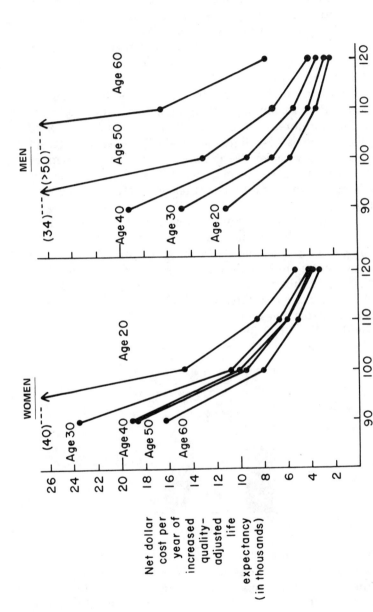

Figure 8-2. Estimated cost effectiveness of treating hypertension, by sex, age, and pretreatment diastolic blood pressure, and assuming full adherence to therapy. (*Source:* M. Weinstein and W. Stason, Allocation of resources to manage hypertension, *New Engl. J. Med.* 296:732–739, 1977. Reprinted, by permission, from *The New England Journal of Medicine*.)

cost-effectiveness ratios approximately double—from $10,000 to $20,000 for patients with mild hypertension and from about $5,000 to $10,000 for those with more severe hypertension (Figure 8.3). Nonadherence, therefore, is a factor to be reckoned with in making clinical decisions.

Other results of our analyses indicate that it is often a better use of resources to attempt to improve adherence of patients who are already under care than to conduct public screening to identify more hypertensives. Furthermore, they indicate that workup for causes of secondary hypertension is best done selectively, for example, screening of patients for renovascular disease with intravenous pyelograms or renograms can be reserved for patients in whom the diagnosis is strongly suspected or whose blood pressures are difficult to control with medications.

How can results of this kind be used? First, they can be used by physicians to help set priorities in their own practices; for example, to guide the allocation of their time between different patients. Time spent with a busy young man with a high diastolic BP who has had difficulty adhering to his regimen because his regimen of taking medicine four times daily interferes with his work day would, very likely, represent a better investment of time than that with a sixty-year-old man with a BP of 180/95.

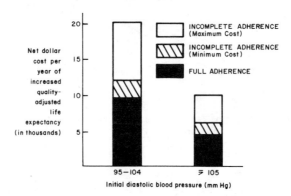

Figure 8-3. Effects of alternative adherence assumptions on the cost effectiveness of treating mild hypertension (diastolic blood pressure of 95 to 104 mm Hg) and moderate or severe hypertension (105 mm Hg and above). Results are for forty-year-old subjects. The analysis assumes age-varying partial benefit, stepped control, and discounting at 5 percent per year. (*Source:* M. Weinstein and W. Stason, Allocation of resources to manage hypertension, *New Engl. J. Med.* 296:732-739, 1977. Reprinted, by permission, from *The New England Journal of Medicine.*)

Second, results of a study such as this can be used to raise physician awareness of the importance of nonadherence as a cause for the failure of treatment.

Finally, from the point of view of policy, cost-effectiveness estimates can be used to influence decisions about the allocation of resources between possible alternative uses—between hypertension, cholesterol screening, coronary bypass surgery, and CAT scanners, for example. For this purpose, comparable analyses of these other health practices are required. Some are in progress; others, no doubt, will follow. What impact these studies will have remains to be seen.

In our opinion, the major potential of cost-effective decision making for containing health care costs lies not in the direct effects of these analyses on policy decisions, but rather in the daily application of cost-effective principles to decisions by physicians, by hospitals, and by third-party carriers. Enhanced cost awareness, alone, will achieve a great deal. Explicit consideration of the tradeoffs between cost and risks, on the one hand, and benefits, on the other, will achieve even more, both in the direction of containing health care costs and, very possibly, in the direction of improving the quality of care. The challenge is to convince physicians that this is so.

We personally are convinced. Compared to five years ago, my practice has changed considerably. No longer is an intravenous pyelogram a routine part of my workup of a patient with hypertension or an echocardiogram of a patient with an obscure murmur. I doubt seriously if any of my patients has suffered as a consequence. If anything, they are better off because I now spend more time listening to them and working with them on their problems and less time chasing zebras.

But can other physicians be convinced? If so, how? If not, what are the reasons? These are some of the major issues to be addressed.

REFERENCES

1. Weinstein, M. C., and Stason, W. B. *Hypertension: A Policy Perspective.* Cambridge, Mass., Harvard University Press, 1976.
2. Kannel, W. B., and Gordon, T. (eds.). *The Framingham Study: An Epidemiological Investigation of Cardio-vascular Disease*, Section 26. (DHEW Publication No. (NIH) 74–599.) Washington, D.C., U.S. Government Printing Office, 1970.
3. Kannel, W. B., and Gordon, T. (eds.). *The Framingham Study: An Epidemiological Investigation of Cardio-vascular Disease*, Section 30. (DHEW Publication No. (NIH) 74–599). Washington, D.C., U.S. Government Printing Office, 1974.

Chapter 9

The Role
of Physician Education
in Cost Control

*Robert S. Lawrence**

The 1976 estimate for the cost of health care in the United States amounted to 8.6 percent of the gross national product. For example, in 1975 more than $4 billion was spent in Massachusetts alone for health care that amounted to 10.5 percent of the gross state product. The sharp increase in expenditures for health stimulated the preparation of the "White Paper on Health Care Expenditures in Massachusetts" by the Health Planning and Policy Committee of the Commonwealth.[1] This otherwise informative document makes no reference to the role of physician education for cost containment, focusing instead on the regulatory functions of state government with a few words about health education and primary prevention. This lack of reference to the education of physicians is reflected in the paucity of information available from the medical literature. If it were not for the contributions of Steven Schroeder, John Eisenberg, and Mohan Garg, there would be almost no empirical data about the relationship of physician education to cost containment.

In recollecting the teaching I had received as a medical student

*Director, Division of Primary Care and Family Medicine, Harvard Medical School.

about the cost of medical services, I only remember a wise senior physician asking me on visit rounds what I planned to do with the serum chloride I had ordered for one of my patients. After confessing that I had no particular plans for that datum I was then asked how much I thought this unnecessary test had cost my patient. I, of course, had absolutely no idea. More typical of the content of clinical education is the following attending note written about a patient with documented extrinsic asthma recently admitted to one of the Harvard teaching hospitals:

> The most likely diagnosis, despite age, is extrinsic asthma. Therapy should be conventional with steroids, bronchodilators, hydration and possibly sedation, with special emphasis on high dose steroids acutely until symptoms are reversed. Then, Cromolyn trial should begin. It is imperative, however, to ruleout occult causes of intrinsic asthma to include: occult recurrent pulmonary emboli, Ascaris or Strongyloides infestation, carcinoid, and, most especially, occult recurrent left ventricular failure (? atrial myxoma; ? old cardiac trauma). To this end, though yield is likely to be quite low, I'd suggest: 1) stool for O&P, 2) urine 5 HIAA, 3) ECHO (R/O LA myxoma); ESR (especially with history of prior lowgrade temperatures, 4) sputum for AFB culture and smear—also fungal culture and smear for possible allergic aspergillosis, 5) finally, though yield is likely to be low, the distinction between allergic bronchitis and/or primary atypical left ventricular failure cannot be made until a trial of a cardiotonic regimen is made. Some consideration should be given to a short course of digitalis and/or diuretic during this hospitalization. If there is seeming improvement, this impression can be firmed up by exercise testing.

It is not surprising that the typical medical student has limited knowledge of costs of medical care and develops attitudes that place undue emphasis on the indiscriminate use of diagnostic procedures. In the same manner that we attempt to deny our own mortality, most medical students and house officers are trained as though we can triumph over all uncertainty in clinical decision making. Skipper and colleagues observed that the liberal use of the laboratory stems from the physician's desire to establish baseline data and avoid litigation and from the physician's lack of information about the costs of tests.[2] To document the latter assumption they selected thirty-one commonly used laboratory tests and asked students, house officers, and faculty at the Medical College of Ohio at Toledo to estimate the costs. Of the sixty-one respondents, 34.6 percent had good knowledge, defined as within plus or minus 25 percent of the actual cost; 38.2 percent gave low estimates, and 27.2 percent gave high estimates. The percentage of good estimates ranged from a low of 27.6 percent for first-year students to 44.6 percent for clinical faculty. As the students progressed through school their knowledge of the costs of diagnostic tests increased slightly, accompanied by a marked shift from overestimates of costs to underestimates. Roth studied forty physicians practicing in a 500-bed community hospital and found only 13.6 percent of estimated costs to be accurate.[3] Forty-one percent of the estimates were too high and 45 percent were too low. Thirty-two of the physicians underestimated aggregate billings for the twenty-two test items by almost 20 percent.

The lack of knowledge of health costs has been accompanied by a change in physicians' attitudes toward costs as government programs and insurance plans buffered the relationship between patient and doctor. The portion of the hospital visit or medical procedure paid directly out-of-pocket declined from 52 percent in 1965 to 33 percent in 1975.[4] During the same period the public share of total health costs increased from 26 percent to 42 percent, making it easier for the physician to do what he or she thinks is best for his or her patient regardless of the cost. Yet only seven years ago Bates and Mulinare were describing the reluctance of physicians to order "ideally" desired tests because of the expense for their patients.[5]

Having mentioned knowledge and attitudes, I would like now to discuss physician behavior. Pineault studied the behavior of thirty-four internists practicing in the Kaiser Portland Health Plan.[6] He found that the physicians who had trained in university teaching hospitals were conservative in their use of laboratory and technical resources when diagnostic ambiguity was low but became more liberal than their colleagues who had trained in community hospitals when the ambiguity increased. Sixteen of the internists had subspecialty training, and this group used more technical resources than the eighteen nonspecialists. Among all physicians variation in the use of technical services was highest for chronic disease and lowest for acute disease. Older physicians were lower utilizers of laboratory services than younger physicians, but there was no relationship between patient load and laboratory use. How much this age association represents imprinting during periods of intense training versus clinical maturity needs to be studied.

In a study of eight internists in group practice Lyle noted wide variations in office productivity.[7] He noted that some physicians recycled their patients more frequently with a much higher proportion of physician-initiated visits. These physicians also tended to have patients with longer hospital stays, and a higher percentage of their patient encounters led to hospital admission. The effects on the health care system of such behavior are that fewer patients obtain service and the cost for those receiving care is disproportionately high. Lyle observed, "Financial incentives to the physician himself may have little bearing on his behavior. It is theoretically possible to generate as much income by having a high number of encounters with individual members of the small patient pool as it is to have a lower number of encounters with a larger pool of patients." Freidson observes that the primary practitioner "gradually builds up a stable lay clientele by a process of client selection; those who do not care for his ethnicity, background, location, hours, personality, manner, and therapeutic and diagnostic prejudices do not return after a trial visit."[8] The patients who continue to come have selected a physician with characteristics and practices that satisfy them. Thus, some of the patterns documented by Lyle may reflect accommodations to the shared characteristics of patients and doctors who feel more comfortable with frequent encounters. Hardwick and associates asked a stratified sample of eighty Canadian physicians to solve a simulated patient management problem.[9] Their assessment revealed a great variety in physician decision-making strategies reflecting numerous phenomena: differences in experience, background, and training; and differences in places of work, available facilities, and nearness of experts and technical personnel. The authors cautioned against developing any general scheme of restraint on medical diagnostic procedures because of the observed differences in clinical problem-solving behavior. Spitzer broadened this approach and presented nine clinical situations to physicians and students at the teaching hospitals of McGill University.[10] He found that for each clinical situation the physicians stratified into three groups: (1) those who would always order a certain test regardless of its cost; (2) those who would never order a certain test no matter how inexpensive it was; and (3) the cost-conscious physicians who would allow the cost of the test to influence their decision about ordering it. The insurance status of the patients in the clinical situations had little effect on physician tendency to institute investigations on the basis of clinical judgment alone, on the one hand, or with sensitivity to costs of the test, on the other hand. The students and physicians were also asked to report the frequency with which the financial implications of laboratory procedures were discussed by attending staff with students at various levels. Thirty-eight percent of the medical students, 30 percent of the interns, and 22 percent of the residents reported having discussions of the cost implications of laboratory tests within the previous week. More than 80 percent of both teachers and learners reported such discussions within the previous six months. The respondents were also asked whether they would favor a laboratory reporting system that included the costs of the procedures along with the results. About 75 percent of respondents favored such a system with 20 percent opposed. However, when asked whether they would favor a reporting system that tabulated the cost of tests ordered by each physician on a monthly or quarterly basis, just under 50 percent were in favor. The most striking result of the study was the finding that regardless of the career stage of the students and physicians, about half of the decisions to order laboratory tests or other investigative procedures were taken on clinical grounds alone without consideration of cost factors. There were no clear trends of increasing or decreasing cost consciousness from students to residents to staff physicians. Spitzer concluded that educational determinants have very little effect on patterns of investigative activities undertaken by physicians. Cost consciousness appears to be a minor factor and unpredictable, a basic personality trait, perhaps like type A and B and amenable only to intense behavior modification techniques.

Other studies suggest that cost consciousness can influence physician behavior. Schroeder and colleagues studied thirty-three internists at George Washington University and noted a seventeenfold difference in laboratory use and a fourfold difference in drug prescribing among this group.[11] After distributing the results of the cost audit, they observed a 29.2 percent decrease in laboratory costs and a 6.4 percent increase in drug costs. Eight physicians in the group sought out the investigators and inquired about the cost profiles. This group had a greater decrease in laboratory cost and combined costs than was observed in the remainder of the group who made no inquiry about their profiles. I believe this group would belong to the cost-sensitive cohort in the Spitzer dichotomy of physician behavior.

These salutory changes in physician behavior appear to be short-lived, however. At the Philadelphia Veterans' Administration Hospital, Eisenberg studied the utilization of prothrombin time determinations by sixty-nine house staff on the study service and forty-five on the control service.[12] A six-week educational program was conducted on the study service to encourage the house staff to reconsider their use of the prothrombin time. Repeat of audits of both services showed a significant decrease in the use of the test on the study service to a low of 55 percent six months after the educational program. In contrast, the control service utilization increased to a peak of 98 percent. No further educational program was carried out for either service during the next twelve months, and the use of prothrombin time determinations by the study service gradually returned to the preeducation levels. In discussing these findings, Eisenberg observes that "modification of clinical behavior should be repetitive to be lasting. It is a well-known principle of behavior modification that behavior is most easily and effectively changed if the stimulus for change is repeated. Second, it is possible that if incentives had been offered to the house staff, the change in their behavior would have been more rapid, more profound, or more lasting. The potential influence of incentives is suggested by a second principle of behavior modification: responses are likely to occur more often if they are followed by rewards (conditioning) and to decrease if they are consistently unrewarded (extinction) or punished."

Dixon and Laszlo tried a different approach toward modifying physician use of laboratory tests. Charts were selected at random from patients of the Durham VA Hospital and the number and type of clinical chemistry tests were recorded.[13] A subjective assessment was then made as to how often clinical chemistry data altered the course of patient care. Only five percent of studies appeared to influence patient care. Each intern on the study ward was then limited to eight tests per patient per day, and subsequently the percentage of chemistry determinations that altered patient care increased to 23 percent. Prior to the limitation six tests per patient per day were performed, and this decreased to two tests per patient per day after the limitation was imposed. The overall reduction of the daily workload of laboratory was 25 percent. Unlike Eisenberg's study, no data were collected to document the long-term effects of the Dixon-Laszlo maneuver.

Before placing undue emphasis on the cost of excessive laboratory tests, it is worth reviewing the other ways in which physician behavior determines the cost of medical care. In 1976 an estimated $120.4 billion were spent on personal health services in the United States, of which 77 percent or $93 billion were generated by practicing physicians in three major sectors: (1) hospital care (including the decisions to admit patients, advise elective procedures, and determine time of discharge); (2) direct physician services; and (3) prescription of drugs and other medical supplies.

In a recent study by the National Blue Shield Association, Carels divides these three areas into eleven inflationary cost factors directly attributable to physicians.[14] They include:

1. New medical technology
2. Drugs and pharmaceuticals
3. Number of laboratory and x-ray procedures done
4. Conflict of interest when physicians own expensive equipment
5. Specialization of medical education
6. Increase in ratio of physicians to population
7. Physician training that emphasizes "technological imperative" rather than allocation of limited resources
8. Physician unawareness of cost implications of their decisions
9. Defensive medical practice
10. Reimbursement mechanism for hospital radiologists and pathologists
11. Trends in medical practice that go beyond saving life and attempt to improve it

In order to decide on the most effective uses of educational resources (or financial incentives, government regulations, or any other approach to cost containment), sensitivity analyses should be applied to these eleven factors to predict the greatest impact on total cost for any reasonable percentage reduction in expenditure for each factor. In other words, since drug costs are 9 percent of total personal health costs compared with hospital care at 46 percent of total costs, influencing physicians to use drugs more appropriately would have less impact than influencing physicians to eliminate unnecessary hospitalizations. At present, data are insufficient to permit detailed sensitivity analyses in many of these areas. These data are urgently needed.

Even more elusive to quantify are the costs attributable to iatrogenesis, whether to the hospitalizations precipitated or prolonged by adverse drug reactions, errors in diagnosis or management, or to the opportunity costs for patients experiencing iatrogenic disability. Illich goes one step further in his assertion that the lay public has been systematically stripped of its ability to provide self-care, a commodity considerably less expensive than physician services.[15]

We seem to be left with the observation that physician cost sensitivity is part of a basic behavior pattern that may prove as immutable as smoking, excessive eating, or the failure to wear seatbelts. Furthermore, the variations among physicians in their sensitivity to costs is matched by a complex health care system with multiple factors influencing costs, all of which is set against the backdrop of a society that has never distinguished itself in resource allocation. Without some change in financial incentives or governmental regulatory function, physicians are no more apt to limit medical expenditures than they are to correct geographic and specialty maldistribution by themselves. Nonetheless, I would be remiss in not making some recommendations about the role of physician education in cost control.

First, cognitive material about the costs of laboratory and x-ray procedures should be included in the curriculum along with instruction about medical economics at the micro and macro levels. Use of peer review and quality assurance audits should be encouraged at the student and house staff level, as well as for practicing physicians, with appropriate emphasis on efficiency and cost effectiveness as integral standards for measuring quality.

Second, there should be greater emphasis in the medical curriculum on attitudinal factors. Students and house officers must be encouraged to recognize and accept a measure of ambiguity and uncertainty in clinical decision making and to adapt probability theory to clinical decision making under conditions of high uncertainty. Perhaps in this way the driving power of the technologic imperative can be blunted.

Third, the clinical settings in which medical education occurs should be expanded to provide a more realistic "patient mix" for students and house officers. In his classic paper on the ecology of medical care, Kerr White noted that for every 1000 people in one month's time there were 750 sickness episodes that stimulated some action on the part of the ill person; 250 episodes generated a visit to a physician, which in turn led to seven hospital admissions, only one of which was referred to a teaching or tertiary care hospital.[16] Yet virtually all clinical education occurs around this one patient in a thousand. Such patients are often critically ill and require the full resources of the modern tertiary care hospital with its angiography suite, CT scanner, and SICU, MICU, and RICU. In this setting the student and house officer can, and usually do, become proficient in diagnosing and managing illnesses that were uniformly fatal several decades ago. But this very same setting is unhospitable to the development of skills in and favorable attitudes toward the techniques of talking and listening rather than manipulating and measuring. Unless more opportunities are available for students to learn from patients in ambulatory settings where common problems are presented in greater variety, where ambiguity rather than technical precision dominates, and where chronic diseases stemming from the interplay of hereditary endowment, personal habits and family and environmental stresses tend to frustrate rather than feed into the physician's rescue fantasies, the process of medical education will contribute little to cost containment.

REFERENCES

1. White Paper on Health Care Expenditures in Massachusetts. Health Planning and Policy Committee, Department of Public Health, Commonwealth of Massachusetts, Feb. 1977.
2. Skipper, J. K., Smith, G., Mulligan, J. L., and Garg, M. L. Physicians' knowledge of cost: The case of diagnostic tests. *Inquiry*, 13:194-198, 1976.
3. Roth, R. B. How well do you spend your patients' dollars? *Prism*, Sept. 1973.
4. Tosteson, D. C. The rising cost of medical care: A doctor's dilemma. *Chicago Med.*, 79:1146-49, 1976.
5. Bates, B., and Mulinare, J. Physicians' use and opinion of screening tests in ambulatory practice. *J.A.M.A.*, 214:2173-80, 1970.
6. Pineault, R. The effect of medical training factors on physician utilization behavior. *Med. Care*, 15:51-67, 1977.
7. Lyle, C. B., Applegate, W. B., Citron, D. S., and Williams, O. D. Practice habits in a group of eight internists. *Ann. Int. Med.*, 84:594-601, 1976.
8. Friedson, E. *Professional Dominance: The Social Structure of Medical Care.* New York, Atherton, 1970.
9. Hardwick, D. F., Vertinsky, P., Barth, R. T., Mitchell, V. F., Bernstein, M., and Vertinsky, I. Clinical styles and motivation: A study of laboratory test use. *Med. Care*, 13:397-408, 1975.
10. Spitzer, W. O. Educational determinants of paraclinical investigation by physicians in teaching hospitals. Paper presented to the Association of Canadian Teaching Hospitals and the Association of Canadian Medical Colleges at their Annual Meeting, Vancouver, B.C., Oct. 5, 1976.
11. Schroeder, S. A., Kenders, K., Cooper, J. K., and Piemme, T. E. Use of laboratory tests and pharmaceuticals—variation among physicians and effect of cost audit on subsequent use. *J.A.M.A.*, 225:969-973, 1973.
12. Eisenberg, J. M. An educational program to modify laboratory use by house staff. *J. Med. Ed.*, 52:578-81, 1977.
13. Dixon, R. H., and Laszlo, J. Utilization of clinical chemistry services by medical house staff. *Arch. Intern. Med.*, 134:1064-67, 1974.
14. *Professional Relations Manual, 1977.* Chicago Blue Shield Association, 1977.
15. Illich, I. *Medical Nemesis: Expropriation of Health.* New York, Random House.
16. White, K., et al. The ecology of medical care. *N. Engl. J. Med.*, 265:885-892, 1961.

Recapitulation

John Gordon Freymann*

I would like to summarize what I think are the most important ideas expressed during this conference. But before discussing them I must remind you that the high cost of medical care is a multifactorial problem and is not going to be solved by simple solutions. Simple solutions will inevitably be complicated by a rough economic analogue to Newton's law: To every action there is often an equal and opposite reaction. For example, we heard that improving the quality of care by cutting down injections in one rural state lowered physician income so much that it led to a decline in the number of practitioners who will accept Medicaid patients. Dr. John Millis puts it another way in what he calls the Principal Principle: "Solutions are the cause of all our problems." One example of the Principal Principle is the looming surplus of physicians. It is the result of a great national effort to solve a physician shortage. It was one hell of a solution—it really solved that problem! But this new problem is going to be with us through at least the first quarter of the twenty-first century.

The basic theme of this conference is that what physicians should strive for is not cost containment but *appropriate care*. Cost containment is a negative concept. Appropriate care is a positive concept, and people prefer something that is positive. These two words,

*President, National Fund for Medical Education.

"appropriate care," connote a great deal. First of all, they connote that we must know how effective specific diagnostic and therapeutic interventions really are. The words also connote that we must know the setting where the care is best delivered—in hospital, office, home, or workplace—and by whom the care can be rendered most effectively—physician, allied health professional, patient, or family. Finally, the words "appropriate care" carry no connotation that quality and cost are necessarily related.

Three points of attack have come out of our discussions. First, the public. We must convince the public that the quality of medical services is not necessarily proportional to the price and that the best kind of medicine does not always involve doing something. Often the patient judges quality by whether the physician is "doing something," e.g., ordering more tests or writing a prescription for an antibiotic or a tranquilizer. Americans have traditionally subscribed to the aphorism "Don't stand there; do something!" In many instances this should be turned around to "Don't do something; stand there!" (This might also apply to Congress as it tries to solve our problems for us.) Another idea that we need to get over to the public is that pressing malpractice suits will not necessarily make medical care better. In fact, excessive litigation has probably had the opposite effect by stimulating defensive medicine and the inappropriate use of medical resources.

The second point of attack is the third-party payers. Two problems came out in this conference. One is that third-party payers currently offer economic incentives that tempt physicians to increase their use of diagnostic tests. The second and probably more important one involves the economic incentives that drive patients into inappropriate and more expensive settings for care. A case in point is the failure to reimburse, or reimburse inadequately, for treatment provided in an office while the same services are reimbursed fully when they are provided in an emergency ward or hospital bed.

The third point of attack is physicians themselves. A number of ideas were developed. One is appropriate use of consultations. When I was a Fellow at the Mayo Clinic I was regarded as rather weird because I like to look at patients' eyegrounds. The routine at the Mayo Clinic at that time was to refer all patients to ophthalmology to have their fundi examined. The same principle is still applied in many residency programs: pelvic examinations are supposed to be done by gynecologists, skin rashes are referred to dermatologists, and so on. If we can teach all physicians—not just primary physicians, but all physicians—not to go into shock when they see poison ivy and to be able to do a pelvic examination and be reasonably sure of their findings, we can save enormous amounts in both direct and indirect costs. As Dr. Eisenberg pointed out, the latter includes the cost to the patient and to the national economy of the time lost in obtaining medical services.

Another factor that is seldom considered is what Dr. Lyle has called "cycling"—how often the doctor has the patient return for follow-up visits. Here again, both direct and indirect costs are involved. Teaching communication techniques to doctors—teaching doctors how to teach patients—is another key area that has enormous cost implications. Failures in patient compliance cause waste. Effective communication with patients is a prerequisite to compliance, and it also minimizes the risk of malpractice suits.

Finally, we come to what I think is the most important point: the way physicians use resources—what Duncan Neuhauser and Bill Stason called "cost-effective clinical decision making." This should be applied to all diagnostic and therapeutic interventions. But can cost-effective clinical decision making be taught? Dr. Lawrence raised this question. Maybe it can't; maybe there is some innate quality in physicians that makes them unable to accept this way of reasoning. If that is so, we should find out. There has never been any research done on this, despite a great deal of research aimed at what makes a medical student a good doctor. If effective research can be done in such an esoteric area as defining doctors' level of moral reasoning (this is now underway at the University of Connecticut), research on the ability of physicians to employ cost-effective clinical decision making should be relatively easy. If specific qualities can be identified, then it should be possible to select medical school applicants who have cost-effective clinical decision making built into their personalities. This is a mind-boggling concept, but perhaps it should be considered.

But I am not that pessimistic. I think we *can* teach cost-effective clinical decision making. I have three reasons for believing this. First, we've never tried to teach it before. Physicians' ignorance of this principle is abysmal. The vast majority of physicians, both those in practice and those now in training, have no concept of cost benefit and cost effectiveness. Instead they have a naive security in numbers, whatever the source or reliability of the figures, which probably devolves from the excessive emphasis on quantitative science in the early years of their education. A number gives them something they can hang onto, so-called pseudo-quantitative medicine. Many factors important to clinical decision making—such as the history, physical examination, and the patient's body language

—can't be quantified, but proper use of these kinds of information can be taught, too.

My second reason for thinking that we can teach cost-effective clinical decision making is that we have been eminently successful in teaching *risk*-effective decision making, so much so that few doctors consciously realize that they are factoring the risk to the patient into the probabilities every time they make a diagnostic or therapeutic decision. Finally, doctors quickly learn cost-effective decision making with regard to one resource, *time.* If doctors can learn so quickly to use one resource wisely, why can't we teach them to use another resource—dollars? I think we can, but first we must overcome the difference in the way these two resources are currently perceived. Time is seen as the doctors'; the dollars are not. It's not *their* money that's involved. Their time is valuable; Blue Cross or Blue Shield's money is for somebody else to worry about.

Our biggest challenge is to teach physicians that all the billions spent for medical care *are* their dollars in this sense: since they and only they have the authority to decide how money is spent on diagnosis and treatment, they should be responsible for the way the money is used. The future freedom of our profession hangs on this issue. If doctors do not assume responsibility for the economic consequences of their decisions, then regulatory agencies perforce will. And with that will go our freedom to render what we think is appropriate care of our patients.

List of Participants

John D. Abrums, M.D.   Albuquerque, New Mexico

Carmine Ammiratti   Vice President
                                Professional Affairs
                                Blue Cross and Blue Shield of
                                    Greater New York

Charles S. Amorosino, Jr.   Executive Director
                                Commonwealth Institute of
                                    Medicine
                                Boston, Massachusetts

Robert S. Botnick, M.D.   President
                                Georgia Society of Internal
                                    Medicine
                                Augusta, Georgia

C. Nason Burden, M.D.   Past President
                                Massachusetts Medical Society
                                Taunton, Massachusetts

R. William Burmeister, M.D.   President-Elect
                                Missouri Society of Internal
                                    Medicine
                                St. Louis, Missouri

Thomas W. Cathcart   Vice President
                                Research and Provider Affairs
                                Blue Cross and Blue Shield
                                    of Maine
                                Portland, Maine

Gail Costa

Associate Project Director
Massachusetts Medicaid
   Cost-Effectiveness Project
Boston, Massachusetts

Harold E. Dayton, Jr., M.D.

Houston, Texas

Norman Deane, M.D.

New York, New York

R. W. Dodson

Manager
Professional Affairs Dept.
Medical Service of D.C.
Washington, D.C.

Robert B. Edmiston, M.D.

Executive Vice President
Professional Affairs
Pennsylvania Blue Shield
Camp Hill, Pennsylvania

Hugh S. Espey, M.D.

Quincy, Illinois

George R. Fisher, M.D.

President
Pennsylvania Society of
   Internal Medicine
Philadelphia, Pennsylvania

Coy Z. Foster, M.D.

Dallas, Texas

Laura P. Franciose, R.N.

Director of Provider Professional
   Relations and Utilization
   Review
Blue Cross and Blue Shield
   of Maine
Portland, Maine

T. Reginald Harris, M.D.

Shelby, North Carolina

Louis F. Hayes, M.D.

Vice President
Professional Affairs
Blue Cross–Blue Shield of
   Michigan
Detroit, Michigan

Frank M. Holden, M.D.

Research and Planning
   Coordinator
Veterans Administration Medical
   District No. 1
Boston, Massachusetts

Mark Leasure	American Society of Internal Medicine San Francisco, California
Saul Lerner, M.D.	Chairman Cost Containment Committee Worcester Memorial Hospital Worcester, Massachusetts
Sidney A. Levine, M.D.	Committee on Medical Service Massachusetts Medical Society Boston, Massachusetts
Albert J. Lewis	Director Professional Relations Blue Shield of Rhode Island Providence, Rhode Island
S. N. Mangano, M.D.	Cambridge, Massachusetts
Barry Manuel, M.D.	Belmont, Massachusetts
Donald S. Mayes, D.D.S.	Vice President Dental Affairs Pennsylvania Blue Shield Camp Hill, Pennsylvania
Lawrence C. Morris, Jr.	Senior Vice President Professional Affairs Blue Shield Association Chicago, Illinois
Peter S. New, M.D.	Chairman Practice Management Committee Cape Ann Medical Center Gloucester, Massachusetts
James F. Patterson, M.D.	Chief of Ambulatory Internal Medicine New England Medical Center Boston, Massachusetts
Michael G. Pipito	Director Blue Shield Association Professional Relations Chicago, Illinois
Arthur G. Porporis, M.D.	American College of Radiology Chicago, Illinois

Grant V. Rodkey, M.D.

Vice President
Massachusetts Medical Society
Boston, Massachusetts

Russell J. Rowell, M.D.

President-Elect
Massachusetts Medical Society
Boston, Massachusetts

Marvin J. Shapiro, M.D.

Member of the Board and
    Executive Committee
Blue Shield Association
Encino, California

William C. Stronach, J.D.

Executive Director
American College of Radiology
Chicago, Illinois

William H. Todd, M.D.

Long Beach, California

Dana Wickware

Staff Editor
Patient Care Magazine
Darien, Connecticut

William M. Wilder, M.D.

Shreveport, Louisiana

Sankey Williams, M.D.

University of Pennsylvania
Philadelphia, Pennsylvania

Gordon D. Winchell, M.D.

Lincoln, Massachusetts

James M. Young, M.D.

Director of Medical Affairs
Blue Shield of Massachusetts
Boston, Massachusetts

Conference Speakers

H. Thomas Ballantine, Jr., M.D.
President
Commonwealth Institute of
    Medicine
Boston, Massachusetts

Edward J. Carels, Ph.D.
Director of Research
Health Care Management
    Systems, Inc.
La Jolla, California

Howard Frazier, M.D.
Harvard School of Public Health
Center for the Analysis of Health
    Practices
Boston, Massachusetts

John G. Freymann, M.D.
President
National Fund for Medical
    Education
Hartford, Connecticut

Warren Kleinberg, M.D.
Department of Community
    Medicine
Medical College of Ohio
Toledo, Ohio

Robert Lawrence, M.D.
Director
Division of Primary Care and
    Family Medicine
Harvard Medical School
Boston, Massachusetts

Duncan Neuhauser, Ph.D.

Associate Professor of Health
  Services Administration
Harvard School of Public Health
Boston, Massachusetts

William Rial, M.D.
  (American Medical
  Association)

111 Dartmouth Avenue
Swarthmore, Pennsylvania

Steven Schroeder, M.D.

Health Policy Programs
University of California
San Francisco, California

Mervin Shalowitz, M.D.

Trustee, American Society of
  Internal Medicine
Executive Director, Intergroup
  Prepaid Health Services
Chicago, Illinois

William Stason, M.D.

Associate Professor of Health
  Services Administration
Harvard School of Public Health
Center for Analysis of Health
  Practices
Boston, Massachusetts

Workshop Leaders

George Baker, M.D. — Massachusetts General Hospital
Boston, Massachusetts

Benjamin Barnes, M.D. — Harvard School of Public Health
Center for the Analysis of Health
    Practices
Boston, Massachusetts

George Dunlop, M.D. — Worcester, Massachusetts

John Eisenberg, M.D. — Hospital University of
    Pennsylvania
Philadelphia, Pennsylvania

Jonathan Fielding, M.D. — Commissioner of Public Health
Boston, Massachusetts

Mohan Garg, M.D. — Department of Community
    Medicine
Medical College of Ohio
Toledo, Ohio

Richard Greene, M.D. — Codman Research Group
Washington, D.C.

James Hudson, M.D. — Association of American Medical
    Colleges
One Dupont Circle N.W.
Washington, D.C.

Alvin Mushlin, M.D. — Department of Medicine
University of Rochester School
    of Medicine and Dentistry
Rochester, New York

Heather Palmer, M.D.   Harvard School of Public Health
                                    Boston, Massachusetts

Leon White, Ph.D.   Harvard School of Public Health
                                    Boston, Massachusetts

Discussant:
William Schwartz, M.D.   Tufts University School of
                                        Medicine
                                    Boston, Massachusetts

Index

About the Editors

Edward J. Carels, who received his Ph. D. in psychology from Loyola University of Chicago, is a research and program evaluator for inpatient alcoholism treatment programs at the Comprehensive Care Corporation in Newport Beach, California. Prior to joining the Comprehensive Care Corporation, Dr. Carels served as Director of Research for Health Care Management Systems in LaJolla, California, as a faculty member of Northeastern Illinois University, and as Assistant Vice President of the Blue Shield Association in Chicago. His current research involves the cost-effectiveness of medical care services.

Duncan Neuhauser is Professor of Community Health at the School of Medicine, Case Western Reserve University. Previously, he was a member of the faculty of the Harvard School of Public Health, a staff member of the Center for the Analysis of Health Practices, and a consultant in medicine at the Massachusetts General Hospital. Dr. Neuhauser's research interests include hospital efficiency and cost-effective clinical decision making. He received his Ph.D. in business administration from the University of Chicago.

William B. Stason is a physician trained in internal medicine and cardiology and in disciplines related to health policy and management. He is Associate Professor of Health Policy and Management at the Harvard School of Public Health and a consultant to the Veterans Administration. Dr. Stason's major interests include the application of cost-effectiveness analysis to health practices and health technologies, the evaluation of health behavior and physician-patient interaction as they relate to preventive medical practices and patient compliance, and questions of resource allocation within the health care industry. He received his M.D. from Harvard Medical School and his M.D.H.S. from the Harvard School of Public Health.